"Ioannis Solos has given us a beautiful
of Chinese medicine. He recognizes that
level of cultivation that forms the founda
technique and theory is in service to that. ⌐upporting this perspective
with many sources from the primary literature, he goes on to offer us
practical exercises that may help us cultivate proper intention. This
material will be an excellent supplement to the knowledge of those
whose medical practice is already complemented by training in the
martial arts. Further, it offers those practitioners wishing to learn
qigong a way to do so in the context of their clinical practice. Finally,
Ioannis transmits a deep love and respect for the medicine that is
moving and inspiring. I take this as further evidence that not only is
Chinese medicine flourishing, it has never been doing better."

—*Lonny Jarrett, M. Ac., author of* Nourishing Destiny:
The Inner Tradition of Chinese Medicine

"Ioannis Solos has written a book which deserves to become required
reading for anybody embarking upon a study of Chinese medicine.
The link between acupuncture, Qi Gong and indeed martial arts is
absolute; in this book Ioannis manages to eloquently show how their
unifying principle of cultivating the Spirit is of key importance for
those wishing to take their "needling" skills to a deeper level."

—*Damo Mitchell, author of* Daoist Nei Gong: The Philosophical Art
of Change *and* Heavenly Streams: Meridian Theory in Nei Gong

"Qi cultivation practices are a treasure from China. Many significant Chinese medical physicians, including Hua Tuo, Ge Hong, Tao Hongjing, Sun Simiao and Li Shizhen, emphasized the practice of qi cultivation for their personal health, and to obtain a deeper understanding of Chinese medicine. Ioannis Solos does a superb job of presenting Zhan Zhuang and Yi Quan qi cultivation. He provides a clear, deep and comprehensive teaching about the relationship between qi cultivation and Chinese medicine. I highly recommend *Developing Internal Energy for Effective Acupuncture Practice* to anybody wanting to learn qi gong, tai chi chuan, meditation and energy healing, and especially to acupuncturists. Solos has written an excellent book that brings to life the qi within Chinese medicine."

—*David Twicken, DOM, L.Ac., author of* Eight Extraordinary Channels—Qi Jing Ba Mai *and*
I Ching Acupuncture—The Balance Method

Developing Internal Energy for Effective Acupuncture Practice

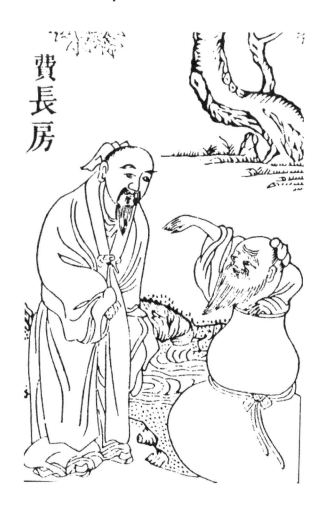

費長房

by the same author

Gold Mirrors and Tongue Reflections
The Cornerstone Classics of Chinese Medicine Tongue Diagnosis –
The Ao Shi Shang Han Jin Jing Lu, and the Shang Han She Jian
Ioannis Solos
Forewords by Professor Liang Rong and Professor Chen Jia-xu
ISBN 978 1 84819 095 5
eISBN 978 0 85701 076 6

of related interest

Heavenly Stems and Earthly Branches—TianGan DiZhi
The Heart of Chinese Wisdom Traditions
Master Zhongxian Wu and Dr Karin Taylor Wu
Foreword by Fei BingXun
ISBN 978 1 84819 151 8
eISBN 978 0 85701 158 9

Eight Extraordinary Channels—Qi Jing Ba Mai
A Handbook for Clinical Practice and Nei Dan Inner Meditation
Dr David Twicken DOM, LAc
ISBN 978 1 84819 148 8
eISBN 978 0 85701 137 4

Daoist Nei Gong
The Philosophical Art of Change
Damo Mitchell
Foreword by Dr Cindy Engel
ISBN 978 1 84819 065 8
eISBN 978 0 85701 033 9

The Compleat Acupuncturist
A Guide to Constitutional and Conditional Pulse Diagnosis
Peter Eckman
Foreword by William Morris
ISBN 978 1 84819 198 3
eISBN 978 0 85701 152 7

Developing Internal Energy for Effective Acupuncture Practice

Zhan Zhuang, Yi Qi Gong and the
Art of Painless Needle Insertion

Ioannis Solos

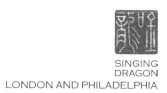

SINGING
DRAGON
LONDON AND PHILADELPHIA

First published in 2014
by Singing Dragon
an imprint of Jessica Kingsley Publishers
73 Collier Street
London N1 9BE, UK
and
400 Market Street, Suite 400
Philadelphia, PA 19106, USA

www.singingdragon.com

Library of Congress Cataloging in Publication Data
Solos, Ioannis, author.
  Developing internal energy for effective acupuncture practice : zhan zhuang, yi qi
gong and the art of
painless needle insertion / Ioannis Solos.
     pages cm
  Includes bibliographical references.
  ISBN 978-1-84819-183-9 (alk. paper)
 1. Qi gong. 2. Mind and body. 3. Acupuncture--Practice. I. Title.
  RA781.8.S64 2014
  613.7'1489--dc23
                          2014000903

British Library Cataloguing in Publication Data
A CIP catalogue record for this book is available from the British Library

ISBN 978 1 84819 183 9
eISBN 978 0 85701 144 2

Printed and bound in Great Britain

"To succeed in this art, you must develop the ability to discover and apply your own fresh ideas, through meticulously reflecting upon the classic theories."

—*Master Cui Fu-shan's Yi Quan guidelines*

In 2002, a very special girl helped me to decipher and appreciate the beauty of Chinese culture. Much of the path I have taken ever since would never have happened without her support, love and guidance all those years ago. This book is dedicated to the eternal memory of Xue Jing-jing 雪晶晶, who was there at the very beginning of this journey.

ACKNOWLEDGMENTS

First of all I would like to thank my teacher, Master Cui Fu-shan, who has bestowed on me true Yi Quan teaching, in accordance with the lineages of Masters Bu Enfu and Yao Zongxun. His ideas and instruction helped me to expand my horizons and develop my imagination in directions I never thought possible. He positively influenced my perception of propriety 德 in the martial, moral, social and energetic sense. He always taught me that "会做人" (which roughly means: getting along with people with decency, dignity and morality) is the highest goal that we should attain as people and martial artists.

Many thanks to Jessica Kingsley, who convinced me to organize and record these ideas on paper. This book would never have been possible without her passion and support.

I am also very much indebted to my very good friends Xue Mei, Liu Meijuan, Zheng Jiazheng, Ryan Bolen, Chen Jiaoling and Megan Williams for all their help and advice during the writing of this book.

CONTENTS

DISCLAIMER   13

PREFACE   15

Introduction   17

PART I ANCIENT CONCEPTS IN THE CONTEMPORARY ACUPUNCTURE CLINIC

1   The Concept of Controlling the Spirit
    (Zhi Shen 治神)   27

PART II YI QUAN EXERCISES

2   Exercise Basics   39
3   The Great Balloon   43
4   Holding the Balloon   51
5   Moving the Balloon   67
6   Acupuncture and Zhan Zhuang   81
7   Training of the Wrist Force
    and Discussion on Other Needling Skills   91
8   Essentials of Zhan Zhuang Practice   105
9   Final Thoughts and Conclusions   115
    BIBLIOGRAPHY   119

PURPLE CLOUD MASTER'S ESSENTIAL METHODS FOR PAINLESS NEEDLE INSERTION

Foreword   124

PREFACE   128

1   Cultivating the Qi   132
2   Training of the Fingers   136
3   Handling the Needle   140
4   Hand Manipulations   142

POSTSCRIPT   146

DETAILED EXPOSITION OF THE INTENTION AND QI EXERCISE

PREFACE   158

1   The Beginnings of Health Cultivation   168
2   The Course of Training
    the Yi Qi Gong Exercise   170
3   Preventing and Eliminating Diseases   184
4   "Intention and Qi Exercise"
    Instructions in Verse   222

APPENDIX 1: MASTER BU ENFU'S YI QUAN
LINEAGE AND TRAINING METHODOLOGY   234

APPENDIX 2: THE COURSE OF THE QI
IN THE INTENTION AND QI EXERCISE   238

ABOUT THE AUTHOR   240

DISCLAIMER

This work has been produced in order to preserve a distinct integration of ancient acupuncture tradition and martial philosophy with the author's unique perspectives on internal training. Neither the author nor the publisher takes any responsibility for any consequences of any decision made as a result of the information contained in this book.

About the translated manuscripts at the end of this book

Translation of pre-modern Chinese texts is a notoriously complicated procedure requiring painstaking efforts and the confrontation of many challenges pertaining to culture and philosophy, cryptic expressions, specialized terminology and even the idiosyncratic expression of the authors. For these reasons, sometimes certain ideas and theories are especially hard to interpret and translate into a Western language.

Therefore, although every effort has been made to ensure that the information in this book is correct, readers should still treat it with caution.

PREFACE

Wang Xiang-zhai was one of the most celebrated teachers of Xing Yi Quan (Form and Mind Boxing) during the first half of the 20th century, and was the last inner gate disciple of the famous Master Guo Yun-shen. Upon his teacher's death, Wang traveled around China meeting famous martial artists, comparing skills and refining his combat understanding. However, at the end of his journey, instead of boasting about the number of techniques he had learned, he did something totally unexpected by modern standards. Wang suddenly dropped all the forms and complicated routines from his teachings and just kept the internal theories. According to Yi Quan lore, he became upset when his early students would pay attention to mastering the external forms, but neglect the cultivation of the intention and mind. Forms, in his opinion, were the external manifestation of a person's mindset, and therefore mind training could potentially totally replace them. The new system was named Yi Quan, meaning "Mind (or Intention) Boxing," and adopted Zhan Zhuang as its core methodology. Theoretically speaking, the various stages of Yi Quan training could guide you step by step towards confidently connecting your mind and body, developing your imagination, and allowing your intention to guide your every move.

How does Zhan Zhuang relate to acupuncture?

The medical classics often speak about the importance of the mind, intention and spirit for the success of acupuncture treatment:

A continuous failure to induce curative effect is due to the acupuncturist's inability to concentrate his spirit essence. When one pays no attention to the mind and intention, his internal and external [harmonies] will be in disagreement, and this will give rise to doubt and may lead to danger. (*Su Wen— Zheng Si Shi Lun*)

The spirit [should] focus on the [needle], and the intention (Yi) should focus on the disease. (*Ling Shu—Jiu Shi Er Yuan*)

Yi Quan, as mentioned above, was developed with a direct focus on how to increase and develop intention, spirit and whole body coordination in accordance with the internal and external harmonies. Therefore, if its training methodology can be modified and adapted to acupuncture training, this can enhance its efficacy.

The basic outline of this book is very simple. Before embarking upon this journey, we should make sure that we have a direct purpose and a destination. The key to this is given in the first chapter. Understanding the concept of Zhi Shen (Controlling the Spirit) will allow us to learn the different skills that we should apply during the various stages of treatment. After these are clearly identified, then we can decide on how best to pursue them in our training. The Yi Quan exercises are presented here in three stages. The first introduces the basic theories needed for building the internal and external connections. The second stage describes how to acquire specific acupuncture skills. Finally, the last stage explains various traditional methods for developing important supplementary skills.

In this book I present my personal opinions, viewpoints and approaches to acupuncture. I hope that my ideas will positively assist others in their journey too.

Introduction

Over the ages, Chinese philosophy, religion, medicine and martial arts have given birth to countless Internal Cultivation traditions. Each of them has its unique flavor, theory, purpose, meaning and sometimes even ritualistic significance within the aspect of Chinese culture that engendered it.

In recent years many such traditions have started to gain popularity in the West. As a result, there are plenty of "Health Exercises" and "Medical Qi Gong" books published in both China and abroad. However, Internal Cultivation texts specifically directed to acupuncturists and "Needling Nei Gong" exercises are rare.

My personal experiences and research

A few years ago, I was learning a family-style Chinese hand-manipulations 手法 modality for tui na in west Beijing. My teacher was initially not very forthcoming with imparting the full system, and for a long time he would cover his hands with a towel during treatment while at the same time trying to evaluate my patience, conduct and personality. However, even though I could not see his form, I noticed that his whole movement strongly resembled a variation of Yi Quan Shi Li. His hand manipulations were soft and powerful, almost effortless, and the patients would feel better as soon as he touched them. His softness and power were a result of his round force 浑圆力 of the whole body, and not of any muscular effort. Later, after he taught me his various healing forms, he urged me to try and enhance my abilities through further personal investigation and self-discovery, and try to work out how to apply these ideas towards improving my acupuncture skills.

During that time I was also living with my Gong Fu teacher and following his exact daily martial workout. One of the most sophisticated skills I learned from Master Cui Fu-shan was his Yi Quan pole theory. Realizing the similarities between Yi Quan pole and needling theory, I had an epiphany that would dictate my acupuncture approaches from that time.

However, I kept meeting other acupuncturists and tui na practitioners around Beijing, and tried to exchange ideas and experiences. One of the recurring themes in their stories was that the old-timers would wake up at 5am every morning and go to the park and practice their calisthenics, every day, regardless of the weather. After finishing their training, they would arrive at the clinic as early as 7am and see their patients. Their touch was very different to the skills we develop today; it was soft and powerful, and could reach deep inside without hurting either the patient or themselves.

These encounters also strongly influenced my way of thinking, because although I was already familiar with martial concepts such as "listening to force," "friction force" and "seeking force," this was the first time that non-martial artists were describing to me the exact same principles and the importance of developing the soft force as a way to protect both the patient and the practitioner.

Hunting for the true Zen Martial Medicine guides

I also think it was during that time that I first came across the term Zen Martial Medicine 禅武医. Apparently, Zen medicine had been scattered and victimized due to political reasons since the Qing Dynasty. Some skills perhaps still survive in the realm of Chinese traumatology and bone setting, but they are mostly fragmentary, and anything of value is transmitted in complete secrecy within closed circles. Being fascinated by this, I tried to learn as much as I could. Again, I started buying rare books, manuscripts and editions of martial guides in the hope that something had survived in the printed literature or was written at the back of a notebook.

Of course, being a Westerner in China did not help much, and people would be even more secretive about such things.

Despite continuous failure to come across a true Martial Medicine guide for acupuncture, I discovered much information about various Cosmic Orbit practices, such as the art of Yi Qi Gong, which is presented at the end of this book.

In modern Traditional Chinese Medicine (TCM) education, the training of Tai Ji Quan and Medical Qi Gong have become quite synonymous with acupuncture. However, in many cases, the way these are taught does not include any specific acupuncture knowledge, except perhaps some meridian and acupoint description. When in the past I briefly taught TCM in the United States, many of my students also told me that their Qi Gong classes were bland and impractical. How can someone progress in the art of acupuncture when the most energetically important classes have no purpose, focus and clinical applicability? Although there is nothing wrong with pursuing Internal Cultivation for general health, longevity and enlightenment, when such a subject is taught as part of an acupuncture course it should at least teach a skill that will be applicable for clinical practice.

Sadly, in recent decades, modern TCM education has placed much attention on becoming a scientifically proven methodology, able to explain everything through neural pathways and the production of endorphins. At the same time it dismisses certain integral aspects of the system, pertaining to cultural teachings, esoteric awareness and psychological and perceptual training. Unfortunately, even after those internal aspects were removed and dismissed as charlatanism, the Chinese acupuncturists still failed to acquire the scientific credibility that they deserved. Even more disturbingly, in certain cases the "simplified" acupuncture also became a healing technique that could be easily taught over a couple of weekends, and adopted by other medical or healing disciplines under different names.

For these reasons, I believe that Chinese acupuncturists should try to practice as closely as possible to the original teachings of the *Huang Di Nei Jing* 黄帝内经 and maintain this mindset, regardless of acceptance issues. Acupuncture research should not focus on one-sided methodologies that place all emphasis on the efficacy of acupoints. Instead they should adopt more integral approaches that utilize the entire system as a whole, and where psychology, rapport, doctor–patient relationship and internal training will be equally addressed in the design.

In any case, even after painstaking research, for a long time I failed to find any pre-modern medical text that exclusively spoke about developing a specific internal skill for acupuncture. At the time I concluded that, although such practices most likely did exist as part of Zen Martial Medicine, they were probably only passed on as teacher–disciple secrets and had been perhaps lost on the way.

The Essential Methods for Painless Needle Insertion

Finally, my breakthrough came in early 2011, when I discovered a rare edition of the *Purple Cloud Master's Essential Methods for Painless Needle Insertion*. This was a short text on developing painless needling, which, in my opinion, also revealed much of the correct attitude and mental training of the competent acupuncturist. The original text was initially discovered and published as "inner-gate" material by Professor Cheng Dan-an in the 1920s, along with his own personal commentaries.

The ideas presented in that short text were amazingly complete, profound and resolute. Holding a true acupuncture internal training guide was a breathtaking experience. The text also strengthened my belief that ancient acupuncturists did have specific training exercises for developing esoteric skills, which were perhaps lost on the way. Unfortunately, even today, a diluted adaptation of painless needling is habitually taught at acupuncture schools without the internal aspects.

After all this excitement, I was eager to provide a translation and interpretation of the original work, and I started researching further and organizing my thoughts and ideas. I felt that an in-depth annotation would allow the modern acupuncturist to fully appreciate the importance of this text. Unfortunately, my priorities changed after 2011 when I started putting together the tongue book *Gold Mirrors and Tongue Reflections*, and as a result I had to let go of the *Acupuncture Nei Gong* work. However, in early 2013, and with the encouragement of Jessica Kingsley, I was happy to go back to basics, reorganize my notes, and start putting things together again.

Nevertheless, although the initial work was originally intended as an interpretation and commentary, it ultimately developed into something totally different which incorporated many of my own personal experiences in China. As I have described previously, for a very long time I was experimenting with my own acupuncture and Nei Gong exercises. The voices of all those people I met during my journey lingered in my mind for a very long time, and eventually the essence of their teachings fused into my daily training regime. Consequently, I developed my own interpretation of several basic Zhuang Fa 桩法 (Standing Meditations) specifically adjusted for training the correct attitude, posture and mindset of the competent acupuncturist. While trying to comment on the Purple Cloud Master's text, these materials kept continuously resurfacing. Finally, I changed the original plan, and instead of writing a commentary I decided to present my personal materials. A translation and photographic reproduction of my copy of the *Purple Cloud Master's Essential Methods for Painless Needle Insertion* is also offered later in this book. I believe that modern acupuncturists can gain much benefit by reading, reflecting and meditating on its words.

Yi Qi Gong

At the end of this book you can find a translation of a second manuscript originally published in 1931, entitled *Detailed Exposition of the Intention and Qi Exercise*, which presents a soft-Kung Fu Cosmic Orbit Healing Meditation called Yi Qi Gong 意气功.

There are several reasons why I decided to include this here. First, I believe that the art of Yi Qi Gong encompasses the same spirit as my exercises, although by application of a very different approach, which demands using the power of the Yi 意 (intention) for circulating the qi over 64 body areas and points in order to induce specific healing effects. This exercise can assist patients with chronic diseases who often relapse and aren't able to frequently visit an acupuncture clinic. With some effort and brief instruction, an energy-aware acupuncture practitioner can teach the patient about this exercise, and how to effectively use it as a supplement to the treatment.

Second, I think that the ancient tradition of Yi Qi Gong has all the attributes that the modern art of Medical Qi Gong originally wished to include in its core in the 1950s. However, it appears that the direct link of Yi Qi Gong to Taoist and Buddhist practices was probably less attuned to the ideology of the realm.

Third, I also wanted the original text to be included here as a training routine for all new acupuncture students who wish to explore and experience the movement of qi in their body, and the function of specific acupoints in restoring balance and health.

Why is this practice important?

Much of the content of this book is an advanced guide explaining what I believe to be some of the most refined skills that someone should try to develop during their career as an acupuncturist.

As an acupuncturist you de-facto deal with energies. Since patients are in principle receptacles of negative energies and stagnations, there is a high probability that some of this negativity will be passed on to you. You have probably noticed how sometimes new acupuncturists and tui na practitioners feel exhausted after merely seeing a couple of patients. The way to deal with this situation is by increasing your internal energy (prior to treatment), becoming able to shield yourself from the negativity (during treatment) and purging all the residual negative energies (after treatment). In this way you can cultivate your health while ensuring that you can provide successful healing throughout your working day, maintain your balance, and also avoid being insulted by your patients at the energetic level.

In addition, regardless of whatever manipulation you use, the ancient books uphold that the most important skills in acupuncture are controlling the spirit and applying intention to your needling. When you can efficiently employ such skills, every manipulation will bring the desired effect. This is because 90 percent of acupuncture first happens mentally, and also because for it to work you first have to truly believe in what you do.

Achieve great things through hard work

Acquiring Nei Gong skills differs from other disciplines, because it doesn't come from reading numerous books, cross-referencing and classroom teaching with discussion. Instead it derives from meticulous hard work, step-by-step self-realization, and correct focus on the skill that you seek to develop. Guidance and learning require a teacher, but unfortunately even the best instructor cannot replace hard work and daily training, without which the skill will never flourish.

The ancient Chinese used the expression 劳苦功高 (láo kǔ gōng gāo), literally to describe someone who achieves great things through hard work and bitter experience. Keep this in mind, especially if seeking to develop any skills through Internal Cultivation.

How to use this book

If you have just started learning acupuncture and you have no Chinese Internal Martial Arts training, I suggest that you begin by contemplating the theory of Zhi Shen (Controlling the Spirit) and discover how to approach each patient. Energetically, I strongly advise that the best way to learn is through seeking a real teacher who can instruct you properly in the basics of Cosmic Orbits, Tranquil Sitting and also Zhan Zhuang. When you understand the important principles, you can try performing the rest of these exercises.

People with previous Chinese Internal Martial Arts training, or Zhan Zhuang meditation experience, can start directly with the Zhan Zhuang exercises.

When performing the Zhan Zhuang exercises with a needle, always be aware that you train for puncturing a patient. Never perform extremely large movements, and always be aware that the needle should not move too much. Visualizing having a patient in front of you will make your training more realistic and applicable.

Always be careful and keep in mind the words of the *Huang Di Nei Jing*:

> When an acupuncturist is needling, his form should be as if he's standing beside an abyss, the hand [holding the needle] as if grabbing a tiger, and the spirit should not be disturbed by anything else. (*Su Wen—Bao Ming Quan Xing Lun*)

I have attempted to write this book in a very simple and concise manner. I wanted to include all the essential instructions while keeping a distance from detailing much of the mainstream information that can be acquired elsewhere. I hope that, after reading it, you will apply your own thinking and experiences and try to imitate the spirit of what is presented here, rather than the external form.

In conclusion, I hope that all the theories and training methods presented here will ultimately assist modern acupuncture practitioners to acquire the correct attitude in their training, enhance their treatment modalities, and enrich their practice and understanding of Chinese acupuncture.

PART I

Ancient Concepts in the Contemporary Acupuncture Clinic

The Concept of Controlling the Spirit (Zhi Shen 治神)

Acupuncture is a healing art, which traditionally is strongly and inseparably related to the manipulation of the qi. Because it deals with energies at the deepest level, the acupuncturist's job should begin long before one gets to insert the needles, and finish long after the patient has left the treatment room.

This chapter deals with one of the most esoteric ideas in acupuncture, the theory of Zhi Shen 治神 (Controlling the Spirit.)

Zhi Shen in relation to acupuncture is an Internal Cultivation term, which originally derives from the teachings of the *Huang Di Nei Jing*.

This term is made up of two characters, zhi 治 and shen 神. The character zhi in this case is used in the context of 治理 (control) and 调理 (recuperate).

The character shen is made up of two parts: the radical shi 礻 (or 示), which means worshiping; and the character shen 申, which stands for the ninth earthly branch, meaning "to extend" or "to expand." In the oracle bones, the most ancient version of the character, shen appears as depicting a man and a woman having sexual intercourse. The same character is also included within the character dian 電 for lightning, as the outcome of the "intercourse" between heaven and earth. This sense of "closeness," "intimacy" and "joining" as part of the term Zhi Shen will be further explored in this chapter.

In any case, the character shen in Chinese Medicine is most often translated as spirit, although various other authors and scholars also use—among others—the words divinity, psyche, mind and vitality to describe it. In the Chinese tradition, the spirit is central to a whole range of ideas, theories and viewpoints, academic, religious, philosophical, medical and otherwise.

As has been said earlier, acupuncture is not merely an art that places emphasis on the action and combination of the acupoints. Equal importance should be placed on the way that the practitioner interacts with the patient, responds to their emotions and psychology, and acts energetically in order to procure a healing effect. In order to understand how these ideas connect, we should first explore the theory of Zhi Shen before describing the practical exercises that will assist in the positive implementation of the acupuncture needling.

Ordinarily, during the acupuncture treatment, the principle of Zhi Shen permeates the entire healing process, and it is often described as the most important skill that one should develop in order to attain proficiency. The ability to control the spirit is also a criterion used to evaluate the level of the competent acupuncturist.

The *Su Wen* states this very clearly when it says:

> For all kinds of needling, you should first [be able to] control the spirit. (*Su Wen—Bao Ming Quan Xing Lun*)

In general, "controlling the spirit" is the ability of the acupuncturist to maintain complete harmony, balance and focus before, during and after the course of an entire treatment session. This includes:

- maintaining the balance of one's internal and external harmonies

- being able to assess the spirit, mentality and emotions of the patient

- deriving the appropriate treatment strategy based on agile, suitable and logical assessment of the patient's condition (including, besides the physical, also the spiritual and emotional state)

- appropriately using the needles in a way that will induce a therapeutic effect

- inducing a needling sensation, maintaining it and driving it towards stimulating a therapeutic effect

- maintaining the therapeutic effect

- being able to keep one's energetic balance before, during and after inserting the needles

- avoiding disturbances from the environment and needling accidents

- obtaining and maintaining the complete trust of the patient.

In most of the written literature, Zhi Shen is typically explained alongside Shou Shen 守神 (Maintain the Spirit). However, in this book I describe the healing process as divided into four different stages according to several modern views (see references 1, 2 and 3 in the Bibliography at the end of Part II). Every stage is in turn explained in conformity with the skill that should be developed in each case.

Evaluating the state of the spirit before needling (Shen Shen 审神)

The patient has arrived at the clinic, and has taken some time to rest and relax, prior to treatment. At this point, even before they enter the treatment room, you should begin the diagnosis and evaluation of the patient's condition.

The patient's conduct, speech, demeanor, attitude and overall behavior can give some invaluable information about the state of their spirit. These points should be first considered, even prior to observation, auscultation (listening to internal body sounds), interview or pulse-taking.

After you make this assessment, you may be able to obtain a good early indication about the positive or negative outcome of the acupuncture session.

In a very similar way, your spirit will also affect the patient's energies. If you are friendly, polite, understanding, full of good energies and have a decent bedside manner, the patient will feel this positivity resonating deep within their body. This comforting, soothing attitude will help to win the patient's trust, soothe their thinking and initiate the healing process.

These points are examined in the classics as follows:

Therefore, when using the needle, one should examine and observe the patient's bearing (i.e. posture and movement), and identify if the essence (jing), spirit (shen), ethereal soul (hun) and corporeal soul (po) are preserved or lost. If the five [spirits] have already been injured, acupuncture will be unable to provide treatment. (*Ling Shu—Ben Shen*)

The disease of the physical body will definitely harm the spirit. The disease of the spirit will definitely harm the physical body. (*Shen Zhai Yi Shu*)

After this initial evaluation, you should examine the condition of the patient according to channel-differentiation theory, and derive an accurate diagnosis of the disorder. Upon establishing a suitable and intelligent treatment strategy, acupuncture can then be administered safely.

The *Ling Shu* advises about this as follows:

The [correct] method for using the needle demands to [completely] understand the physical form and qi, and their position. Left and right, upper and lower, yin and yang, exterior and interior, and whether [the amount] of qi and blood is sufficient or scanty, [or] if the movement [of qi] obeys or counters [the normal flow]. [If one completely] understands whether the [qi movement] obeys or counters [the normal flow] then they can establish how to best offer treatment. Examine the roots and branches, check about cold and heat (i.e. chills and fever), derive the location of the evil, and acupuncture needling will not cause any harm. (*Ling Shu—Guang Neng*)

Regulating the spirit while inserting the needle (Tiao Shen 调神)

Before inserting the needle, you should be able to control and regulate the spirit. This not only means regulating your own spirit, but additionally you should assist the patient to regulate their own too. This process ensures that the hearts of both you and the patient are calm, your breathing even and your muscles relaxed in order for the qi and blood to flow as unobstructed as possible. Under your initiative, you should both build and maintain some kind of rapport or synchronization in terms of posture, breathing, mutual attention and understanding. After such a link has been established, where trust has been built and both you and the patient feel at ease, it is more likely that the treatment will yield positive results.

The classic texts advise on this as follows:

> If using acupuncture to treat, you should assist the [patient's] spirit to focus and then needle. [This procedure does] not only [apply] for needling but [you should] also allow the [patient's] spirit to become stable before moving the qi. If the spirit is out of focus, then don't needle. If the spirit is stable you can treat [by both needle and moving the qi]. (*Biao You Fu*)

> When needling, the patient's spirit qi must be stable (focused), and his breathing even. The doctor should also do this (i.e. focus and adjust his breathing), and not be hasty. (*Zhen Jiu Da Cheng*)

While administering acupuncture your spirit and the needle should become as one 针神合一. This means that your entire existence and intention 意 should—at the moment of needling—focus on the tip of the needle, and the needle should become an extension of your hand.

The *Ling Shu* says:

> The spirit should focus on one point, and the [spirit] mind concentrate on the [tip of the] needle. (*Ling Shu—Jiu Zhen Shi Er Yuan*)

Of course, this is a skill that needs to be trained. Meditation techniques on developing such a mindset are described elsewhere in the book; however, the classical description is as follows:

> The Tao of grasping the needle requires [one] to firmly hold it like it is a precious treasure. Insert [the needle] with the finger straight [perpendicular], and not angling towards either the left or right. The spirit is at the tip of the needle. Focus on the patient. Be careful to avoid blood vessels, and then needling will bring no harm. (*Ling Shu—Jiu Zhen Shi Er Yuan*)

> When an acupuncturist is needling, his form should be like if he's standing beside an abyss, the hand [holding the needle] as if grabbing a tiger, and the spirit should not be disturbed by anything else. (*Su Wen—Bao Ming Quan Xing Lun*)

Maintaining the spirit after inserting the needle (Shou Shen 守神)

After inserting the needle, you should, through needle manipulation and the power of your Yi-intention 意, try to induce and maintain the therapeutic effect. At this point mental work is required at the deepest level. Your mind should concentrate on two things. First, you should observe the patient closely, and adjust the treatment in accordance to any changes in his spirit and thinking. This is more like a Yin and Yang balancing procedure where, by means of needling and also rapport, you try to assist the patient's recuperation:

> The emperor said: The living person has a form, which does not depart [from the laws of] Yin and Yang. (*Su Wen—Bao Ming Quan Xing Lun*)

> The Tao of grasping the needle requires [one to stand] upright (alt. correctly), and be calm and tranquil. First understand [if the disease is due to] excess or deficiency in order to correctly select fast or slow insertion [or manipulation]. (*Ling Shu—Xie Ke*)

The crude (i.e. the mediocre) acupuncturist maintains the frame; the superior [acupuncturist] maintains the spirit. (*Ling Shu—Jiu Zhen Shi Er Yuan*)

The spirit should focus on one point, and the [spirit] mind concentrate on the [tip of the] needle. (*Ling Shu—Jiu Zhen Shi Er Yuan*)

Second, you should try to achieve the De Qi-Needling sensation 得气, maintain it, and also guide the qi towards the desired direction that will enhance the therapeutic effect. However, this is not an easy feat, and it requires appropriate mental training for developing the ability to concentrate on the patient, adjust the treatment according to the situation at hand, and aim towards inducing a desired effect that will ultimately restore the patient's balance:

The spirit [should] focus on the [needle], and the intention (Yi) should focus on the disease. (*Ling Shu—Jiu Shi Er Yuan*)

During acupuncture, the doctor should visualize as if [he is] staying in a secluded space. He should maintain his spirit, and imagine that all doors and windows are closed to prevent the ethereal and corporeal souls [dispersing]. His intention becomes one with the spirit, essence and qi. [In this mindset] he cannot hear any voices from the outside, so as to accumulate this essence; the spirit should focus on one point, and the [spirit] mind concentrate on the [tip of the] needle. He should apply shallow insertion and retain the needle, or soft and superficial manipulation in accordance with the movement of the spirit. After reaching the qi, he can stop. (*Ling Shu—Zhong Shi*)

The fingers should be like grasping a tiger gracefully and strongly. The acupuncturist should ignore everything that's happening around him and quietly concentrate his mind on observing the patient, while avoiding looking left and right. He should do what is moral and appropriate, and not evil, when inserting the needle: this means that the needle should be held and inserted perpendicularly. The doctor must rectify the spirit: this means that he should gaze into the patient's eyes in order to control his spirit and allow the qi to move [more easily]. (*Su Wen—Zhen Jie Pian*)

Sadly, modern trends in acupuncture training simply demand mere memorization of acupoints and their combination, and do not allow space for proper mental and energetic cultivation. Even in China, most acupuncture schools simply offer the training of watered-down variants of Tai Ji Quan, Ba Duan Jin and other energetic traditions as part of their courses. Although these exercises may be useful for combat and/or general health, in reality they were never designed to achieve the acupuncturist's correct mindset. In my opinion, many good things can be learned from books such as the Tai Ji classics, but in practice nobody teaches any relevant information from these sources in modern TCM education. The empty training of forms cannot replace true internal knowledge and self-discovery. Therefore, only a few dedicated practitioners ever attain higher-level skills, mostly through personal effort.

This reality, combined with ignorance and misplaced trust in trivial modalities, often conveys a negative image of the acupuncturist's character. If the acupuncturist's spirit is scattered, then the effect may cause more harm than good. The *Su Wen* warned about this as follows:

A continuous failure to induce a curative effect is due to the acupuncturist's inability to concentrate his spirit essence. When one pays no attention to the mind and intention, his internal and external [harmonies] will be in disagreement, and this will give rise to doubt and may lead to danger. (*Su Wen—Zheng Si Shi Lun*)

Nourishing the spirit after removing the needle (Yang Shen 养神)

Nourishing the spirit after the treatment is the last part of the healing process. You should be able to regulate your energies, cleanse yourself from negative emotions, and find your balance before resting or moving on to the next patient. It is an important demand that the acupuncturist maintains good health and also a healthy external image, pleasant mood and lively spirits, and that these are reflected effortlessly as an outcome of good health and training, not through acting.

The patient should also be able to maintain their newly restored balance in order to avert the relapse of the disease. Disorder of emotions will strongly affect the internal organs, as is written in the classics:

> Sorrow, grief, sadness and anxiety can trigger the heart to pulsate [abnormally]. The [abnormal] pulsating of the heart will shudder the five zang and six fu organs. (*Ling Shu—Kou Wen*)

Therefore it is prudent that patients become able to regulate their lifestyle, mood and emotions, diet and exercise in order to enhance the therapeutic effect of the acupuncture treatment, and also prevent the disease from forming again:

> The true qi follows tranquility and nihility.[1] If the essence and the spirit are guarded internally, how can illness develop? (*Su Wen—Shang Gu Tian Zhen Lun*)

---

1   In various martial arts traditions this nihility is often termed "the void."

PART II
Yi Quan Exercises

The exercises in this part have a dual purpose. First, they are designed especially for acupuncturists who have had some exposure to Chinese Internal Arts, and especially Zhan Zhuang. The aim is to assist practitioners in building the correct framework, attitude and posture for acupuncture treatment, and also train their intention 意, a vital skill for the correct application of needling.

Second, these exercises are designed to help practitioners maintain a healthy and balanced daily training regime, that can be applicable not only for fitness but also for needling art.

CHAPTER 2

Exercise Basics

A very old Greek folk story tells about a 40-headed dragon that was terrorizing the land. Because the death toll and destruction were overwhelming, the emperor declared that he would share his kingdom with anyone who would slay the dragon and, as a sign of proof, bring back his 40 tongues.

In the end, a knight of the Imperial Guard managed to slay the dragon, and cut off 39 of the tongues. However, because there was a lot of blood, he couldn't find the 40th tongue. But since he had collected 39 tongues he felt that it was already proof enough.

Finally, after the long fight and the cutting off of the tongues, he headed for a nearby forest where he slept under the trees.

Soon after, a peasant who was passing by saw the dead dragon and by pure luck found the missing tongue. He then put it in his pocket and rushed back to the Imperial Palace.

The emperor immediately asked him to show proof that he had slain the monster. The wicked peasant took the tongue out and yelled "One!" Then he put it back in his pocket, pretended to search, and took the same tongue out and cried "Two!"… and so on until he had done it 40 times. The naïve emperor was impressed and decided to share his kingdom with this peasant.

However, while the imperial declaration was being prepared, the knight returned to the palace. He proceeded to present the 39 tongues, begging for forgiveness because he had missed the last one.

The emperor immediately understood that he had been tricked and ordered that the wicked peasant be thrown out.

This old story about a 40-headed dragon and the naïve emperor was used to educate Greek children for many centuries. People kept telling it for two reasons: first, to amuse young children, and second, to educate them about seeing things exactly as they are.

Zhan Zhuang is a very simple type of meditation. To attain proficiency one does not need to learn many complicated routines, or grasp many diverse postures. Especially for health and martial application there is only a handful of postures (in essence only 3–4, but people recognize about 20 variants), all of which have very similar basic external demands.

Their difference is often either the focus of the intention 意 (Yi) or their martial/health application. Therefore, instead of learning many different postures, the student should master several key concepts such as mo jin (seeking forces), the interchangeability of relaxation and tension (physically, mentally and emotionally), and also the six direction forces 六面力, whole body force 浑圆力 and contradictory forces 矛盾力. After one has understood and is able to apply such basic ideas, then any posture will be Zhan Zhuang, and one will have returned to the "natural state," which is the highest level of Yi Quan awareness.

Because of this vital simplicity, anybody who has mastered the internal concepts can adapt any given posture according to their individual needs and intention. This also means that any of the basic postures can have 10 or 100 different variants, but in essence these are merely 100 different faces of the same exercise. People should be wary of this, and avoid anyone presenting them with "1 tongue, 40 times."

This simple fact is exactly what makes the Zhan Zhuang exercises so flexible and able to adapt according to any circumstances. For this reason I have limited all explanations to the essentials, and in accordance with the Yi Quan tradition and philosophy.

Historically, the art of Yi Quan was established only 90 years ago, and since its inception it has taken a very different theoretical path from other old-fashioned Chinese energy cultivation traditions. However, although Yi Quan has its own terminology, in practice many ancient theories (including the dan tian 丹田 [cinnabar field] and the unity of the five elements 五行 and the six harmonies 六和) still survive within the art, but in many instances they are articulated in different ways and as part of a more "holistic" approach.

In the following chapters I will explain some essential principles using modern and traditional terms, in order to assist TCM practitioners with gaining a basic understanding of the art.

However, the way I describe the theories is quite different from the explanations provided in the established Yi Quan literature. Here, I have produced summaries of the fundamentals, broken down into several digestible visualizations. I believe that these may assist practitioners in grasping the concepts easily, quickly and efficiently, even if they haven't been exposed to the complete literature of the art.

I also present these ideas in the hope that my explanations will positively contribute to the popularization of this remarkable meditation tradition.

CHAPTER 3

The Great Balloon

Let's start with a simple exercise, which I call "The Great Balloon," so that I can describe the fundamental Zhan Zhuang theories as part of a whole.

EXERCISE 1: TI CHA ZHUANG 提插桩
External instructions

* Find a peaceful place with plenty of fresh air, away from large crowds, distractions, noises and strong smells.

* Stand with the feet at about shoulder-width apart.

* Slightly bend your knees, with the kneecaps never going further than the toes, and sink your torso as if sitting on an imaginary stand or balloon. Ensure that:

    * your back is straight, your shoulders are down and relaxed, and the chin is parallel to the ground

    * your chest is relaxed and slightly caved in

    * your tongue touches the palate in order to connect the Du and Ren channels separated at birth

    * your hands are hanging at the side, relaxed but not loose, with your palms facing the legs

⟡ you are breathing normally through the nose

⟡ your eyes are looking forwards into the distance.

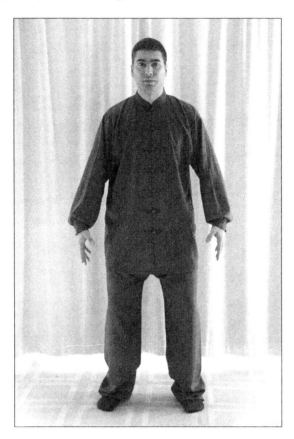

Visualization 1

✦ Imagine yourself inside a great balloon. Its center is your center of gravity.[1]

✦ The diameter of the balloon is your height. This balloon is like a selective field where negative energies cannot enter.

✦ Be flexible about the way you think about and experience these exercises, trying to explore feelings. Don't allow your thinking to become rigid and unyielding.

---

1 "Cinnabar field" (dan tian 丹田).

NOTES

✦ As with any balloon in the physical world, the force of the air pushing the walls outwards is the same as the forces pushing the walls inwards. These exist all around the balloon, and allow it to assume the most energetically stable and efficient shape, much like a drop of water.

✦ The balance of these forces is the simplest paradigm of "contradiction forces" (mao dun li 矛盾力). Just think in Newtonian terms about "every action having an equal and opposite reaction." According to the laws of physics, while being inside the great balloon, if you try to expand—extend your body in any direction—an opposite force from the walls of the balloon will exert its power in order for equilibrium to be maintained.

✦ For example, while your knees are bent, if you try to stand straight, the walls of the balloon will exert an elastic force with the opposite effect.

✦ This visualization will help you to imagine a whole network of internal "rubber bands" that link each part of the body together in order to make it assume the most energetically efficient shape.

✦ In the beginning stages of Yi Quan, we refer to these as the six direction forces, corresponding to a 3D Cartesian axis system. Don't be afraid to explore these forces. Free your mind and try to discover the elastic and opposing forces within your body.

Let's see the mao dun forces in a different way and go back to The Great Balloon exercise.

Visualization 2

✦ Imagine yourself inside the balloon. Its center is your center of gravity. Keep this thought until you feel comfortable inside it and become aware of the six directions of up–down, left–right and front–back.

✦ Next, visualize the great balloon collapsing on your skin, forming a garment that fits your human shape.

✦ However, this garment is very special, because instead of being smooth it contains many hooks and barbed wire which can grab the air, preventing you from moving in the direction you're aiming for.

NOTES 1

✦ This is a different mao dun viewpoint. The internal forces from Visualization 1 still exist within the great balloon that has now taken human shape. After gaining the ability to understand these forces within their new form and shape, you should attempt this exercise.

✦ In this second visualization, the barbed wire and the hooks will prevent large movement in any direction. So if you try to step forwards or backwards, or move any part of your anatomy in any direction, the hooks that face the opposite way will prevent this movement.

✦ Let's add a different thought, too. Imagine that you want to move forwards, but the hooks push you backwards, and then you mentally yield and imagine that you move backwards in the opposite direction. While yielding, the opposite-facing hooks will still push you forwards, and so on. In this way, many cycles are formed back and forth, up and down, left and right, and also diagonally in any direction.

✦ These are also mao dun forces that are supposed to teach you that, for example, within upward movement there is also a downward direction, like many Yin and Yang cycles that never stop moving.

NOTES 2

✦ The visualization with the hooks is used here only for the purpose of understanding the contradictory forces. However, after becoming aware of these, the visualization with the hooks should be discontinued and you should try to explore softer concepts, such as moving while being immersed in water or honey. The same opposing forces also exist in such an environment too, but they allow freedom of movement, which makes them far more applicable in real life.

Finally, there is one more mao dun theory that I would like to discuss here.

Visualization 3

✦ Imagine yourself inside the great balloon. It subsequently collapses, forming the previously mentioned human-shaped garment. This time there are no hooks and barbed wire.

✦ If you are performing this exercise outdoors, try becoming aware of the wind. If you are indoors, imagine that there are winds blowing from various directions.

✦ Allow the wind to pass through the pores of your skin to the other side. Do not let it move you, but allow it to pass through as if you are not solid.

NOTES

✦ This exercise is designed to allow you to experience the mao dun forces in connection with the surrounding environment. You are becoming one with the wind and the surrounding air, you can feel its softness, you are aware of the exact direction of the wind flow, and your inner being becomes one with the qi of the cosmos.[2]

---

2   (a) In the martial aspects of Yi Quan, and at a higher level, the slightest breeze will lead you to adopt a posture that will conform with the direction of the wind, and you will feel like you are becoming "a flag in the wind" or "a fish in the river." The general principle is about finding the least energy-consuming posture in the face of changing circumstances.

(b) The mao dun forces in Yi Quan are also explored in the emotional aspects. Often exercises are devised where, for example, the student has to explore feelings such as anger alongside tranquility. These martial exercises are beyond the scope of this book.

Additional thoughts

At this point we have explored the basic principles of the mao dun li theories. Through the exploration of the contradictory forces you can understand the importance of the six directions, which form the basic directions of 3D Cartesian axes (i.e. with your center of gravity being the center of the axes, the six directions will be right–left, up–down and front–back).

Ultimately, the exploration of all these forces, in every direction imaginable, will lead to the development of the hun yuan li (whole body force 浑圆力), which is one of the highest principles that all Chinese internal martial arts seek to achieve. At that point you become like the flag in the wind, or the fish in the river, as has been described elsewhere.

PRACTICAL APPLICATION: SHIELDING YOURSELF FROM NEGATIVE ENERGIES DURING ACUPUNCTURE ADMINISTRATION
Visualization 4

✦ Imagine yourself inside the great balloon as described above. The balloon eventually collapses, taking the shape of your body, forming an imaginary energy garment.

NOTES

✦ This garment is very selective and prevents the negative energies from penetrating.

✦ Try to maintain the visualization of the balloon throughout your interaction with patients, in order to avoid the exchange of negative energies.

✦ Spirit, form, mind, force and intention, both internal and external, should be unified as one.

+ The four centers should be in harmony (top of the head, dan tian, palm centers and centers of the feet).

+ Make sure that you develop a strong awareness about this imaginative second skin, as this skill will be pivotal in the demands of other exercises.

CHAPTER 4

Holding the Balloon

Yi Quan is popularly associated with exercises such as "Standing Like a Tree" and "Holding the Balloon." Here I continue the traditional sets of exercises by explaining how standing like a tree, holding the balloon and also moving the balloon will assist you in attaining a higher level in your acupuncture practice.

Let's start from the basic standing exercise, and then move forwards.

EXERCISE 2: TUO BAO ZHUANG 托抱桩
External instructions

+ Find a peaceful place with plenty of fresh air, away from large crowds, distractions, noises and strong smells.

+ Stand with the feet shoulder-width apart.

+ Slightly bend your knees, with the kneecaps never going further than the toes, and sink your torso as if sitting on an imaginary stand or balloon. Ensure that:

  ⋄ your back is straight, your shoulders are down and relaxed, and the chin is parallel to the ground

  ⋄ the chest is relaxed and slightly caved in

  ⋄ your tongue touches the palate in order to connect the Du and Ren channels separated at birth

   ⋄ your hands are hanging at the side, relaxed but not loose, with your palms facing the legs

   ⋄ you are breathing normally through the nose

   ⋄ your eyes are looking forwards into the distance.

+ Slowly raise your hands up until they are approximately on the same line with your belly button, as in the photo below.

+ The distance between the hands is about 3–4 fists.

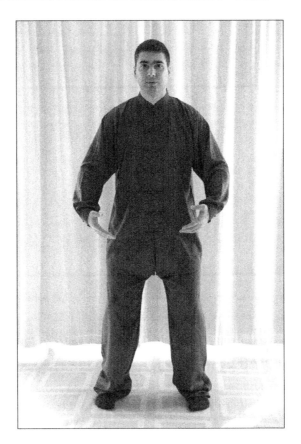

Visualization

+ Imagine that with your arms and your belly and chest you are holding a big balloon. Various others often describe this as Buddha holding his belly.

NOTES

+ In every exercise that demands holding a ball or a balloon, the hands are actually "supporting" and not "holding" the ball, the bottom part of which is always resting firmly on the belly.

+ In this way, the movement of the abdomen (and the core) always dictates the movement of the balloon, while *the hands always follow and never precede the movement of the core.*

+ The mao dun (contradiction) forces are always present.

+ The hands having a supporting role should not exert any physical force on their own, but the force of the core should reach the fingertips. In addition, through the training of the contradiction forces (remember the visualization of the hooks), eventually you will develop from the inside the kind of soft force that is vital in the training of both acupuncture and tui na.

EXERCISE 3: CHENG BAO ZHUANG 撑抱桩
External instructions

+ From the tuo bao zhuang position, raise your hands until they face your chest.

+ The distance between your hands is about three fists.

Visualization 1

+ Imagine that you're still holding the balloon. The hands are there to support the balloon. If they squeeze too much it will pop, but if they are too loose the balloon will fall. Try to work with these contradictions.

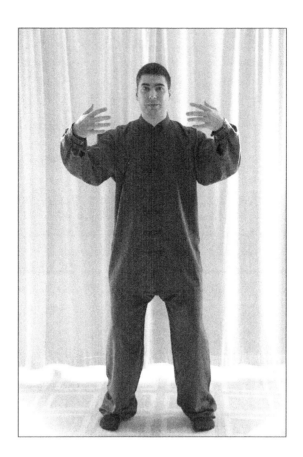

Notes

+ This is the most famous Yi Quan stance, and one of the most important. This is one of the exercises that will greatly assist your understanding of the six directions, and help you best connect your dan tian to your hands, legs and head while energetically strengthening your body from the inside.

Additional visualizations

There are many types of visualization applicable to these exercises, and you can regard each one of them as a totally new exercise. You should also try to adapt them according to your own personal needs. Here I list a few common ones, in accordance with Yi Quan tradition:

✦ Think about being in a pool of warm water up to the waist. Rock your body in any direction, and feel the resistance of the water.

✦ Listen to a distant sound. Try to decipher what it is and where it comes from.

✦ You are in the middle of a storm, with hurricanes and thunder, and with hail falling from the sky. You are like a 2000-year-old tree with strong roots. Nothing can move you.

✦ You are in the shower, and warm water is falling on your body. Relax and let go of all your troubles.

✦ You are in the "great balloon," and its wall is like a metallic spider's web. People throw needles and knives at you. With a whole body movement you move the net and divert their trajectory so they won't hit you.

NOTES

✦ Depending on what you seek to achieve, there is always an appropriate visualization. These can have a medical, martial or some other focus, and in essence they can help—within realistic parameters—your patient and yourself to achieve whatever goal you set.

PRACTICAL APPLICATION: ACTIVATING POINTS AND CHANNELS

Imagine that you are made of dry earth (or sand). There is rain falling on your body, and it gets absorbed inside. You feel like your whole body is thirsty for this water, and each drop reaches deep and quenches your thirst. The rain is made of golden and colorful drops (here you can even add the color of your choice according to Five Elements theory). Each drop is made of positive energies that revitalize you and cancel out all negativity, taking away any mild pain or stress. The rain can either fall on your whole body or just a certain location, according to the effect you wish to induce.

NOTES

Let's review this exercise with a twist:

✦ Become aware of the location on your body of an acupoint of your choice. For this exercise you can imagine a single drop of rain falling on this acupoint and activating its qi. More drops fall, until you realize that the qi of this point can move. The next drop moves to the next point down the channel, and the qi follows. Eventually, if you wish, you can activate part of a channel, or certain points, to achieve a therapeutic effect.

EXERCISE 4: TUI TUO ZHUANG 推托桩
External instructions

✦ From the cheng bao zhuang position, raise your hands to the level of your face.

✦ Turn your palms to face outwards.

✦ The fingers are naturally curved as if they are holding the imaginary balloon.

Visualization

✦ Imagine that you are holding the balloon and you try to push it forwards and upwards. The hands merely support the balloon, but its movement is strictly dictated by the dan tian. Each time you push it, it is the dan tian that pushes it, and not just the fingers.

NOTES

✦ For all of these exercises, the main point is that the work is done mentally and not physically.

✦ If you do these exercises physically your body becomes stiff, while the mental component never gets trained sufficiently.

✦ Most of the Yi Quan teachers called this "the body being relaxed, and the mind tense." This tension is from thinking, and trying to sort out the contradictions. As Master Cui Fu-shan used to say, "In Yi Quan, one has to always think and reflect a lot on each theory and each exercise."

✦ For this exercise specifically, the shoulders often get very tense, especially at the beginning. Try to think about the visualization of the rain. This time, warm rain is falling on your shoulders, taking away the pain and tension with each drop.

✦ Try to keep your frame. To help with this, you can also imagine that you are inside the great balloon and the palms push the wall outwards, while at the same time the feet do the same in the opposite direction. The walls of the great balloon exert the exact opposite force.

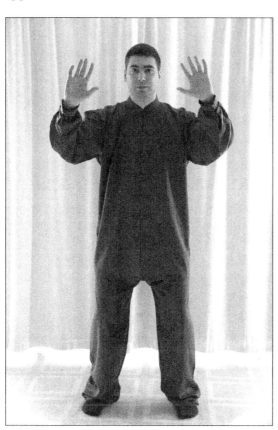

✦ You can also imagine a rubber band connecting the feet with the palms, so each time you push the ball, the opposite force is also felt in your mind.

EXERCISE 5: FU AN ZHUANG 扶按桩
External instructions

✦ From the tui tuo zhuang, slowly lower your hands down to just above the level of the navel.

✦ The fingers are naturally bent and relaxed and pointing forwards.

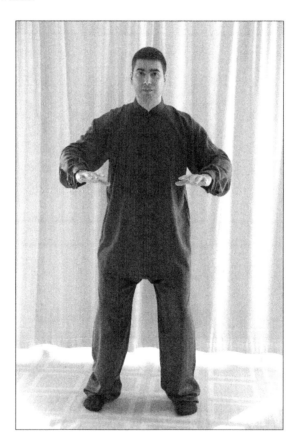

Visualization

+ Imagine that you're standing in the middle of a river, and the water reaches up to the level of your waist. Your hands are resting on a wooden plank or a balloon immersed in the water, and you're trying to adapt your frame in order to resist the forces that are present.

NOTES

+ You can also imagine that your fingers are tied to nearby trees, and that you pull them towards you, or push them away.

+ While in the river you can experiment with the six directions (up–down, left–right, front–back) and see how your body adapts while the water flows or the trees pull you.

+ The entire exercise is done mentally. Try not to tense your muscles too much, and only exert minimum physical force.

EXERCISE 6: XIU XI ZHUANG 休息桩
External instructions

+ From fu an zhuang, slowly lower your hands to fall by your side, as in ti cha zhuang, and then place them at your back, with your he gu (LI-4) touching (or rubbing) your shen shu (UB-23).

Visualization

+ Relax, and think that with your open palms you are holding a paper balloon.

NOTES

+ This is the exercise that you can return to at any point when you get too tired from doing any of the previous exercises.

◆ In many cases, rubbing the shen shu (UB-23) can help you restore some of your energy, especially if as a beginner you have used more the physical rather than the mental to perform these exercises.

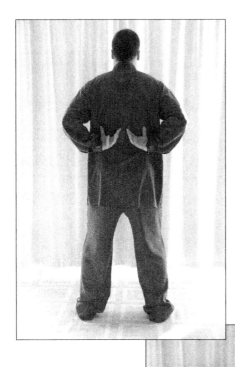

EXERCISE 7: HUN YUAN ZHUANG 浑元桩 VARIANT 1

Hun yuan zhuang is usually referred to as the basic Yi Quan martial stance. While the previous exercises were presented as a prelude to theory, and also for offering a basic balancing training regime, this exercise and the two following ones are more about practical applications. In essence, the same basic principles apply. The three exercises introduce the important ideas that we will later explore in much more depth in the practical applications for acupuncture needling.

External instructions

+ From the cheng bao zhuang position (exercise 3), the right (or left) foot moves forwards for a half step. The back foot turns outwards, forming an angle of approximately 45° with the front foot, and the position of the two feet roughly resembles the Chinese character ba 八. The demands for this foot positioning are that the front foot is not too far forwards, and that there is a comfortable and natural feeling rather than rigidity.

+ The heel of the front foot is slightly raised, as if there is a sheet of paper underneath it.

+ Your weight should be distributed 30 percent on the front foot, and 70 percent on your back foot.

+ The feeling is that your buttocks are sitting comfortably on a giant balloon.

+ Between the arms and the chest there is another large balloon, which your hands are assisting to support in place. Its movement is strictly directed by the dan tian.

+ The pointing finger of the front hand is level with your mouth, and the pointing finger of the back hand is level with the jaw, although this is not a rigid rule.

+ As you look forwards, the tip of the nose, the center of the palm (PC-8) and the big toe of the front foot form an imaginary straight line.

+ As the eyes look forwards, the jaw is parallel to the ground.

+ The distance between the hands is still roughly about three fists.

+ The back of the front hand and the back hand form an imaginary 90° angle between them.

+ Relax the shoulders.

+ The fingers are spread open and relaxed, like holding two paper baseballs.

+ The tongue softly touches the palate.

+ The abdomen is relaxed and round, and the chest slightly drawn in.

+ You should not use any force, but all the movement should be done with the power of the Yi-intention 意.

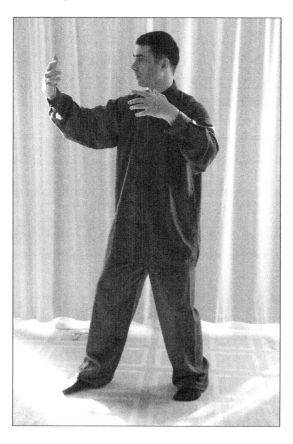

Visualization

+ The earliest visualization for this exercise demanded that the practitioner imagines holding a shield with the front hand and a spear with the back hand. The words mao 矛 for spear, and dun 盾 for shield, were used to introduce the basic martial requirements for this zhuang, but also for the basic concepts of the contradiction forces. The characters for spear and shield put together form the word mao dun 矛盾, which means contradiction.

NOTES

+ This is one of the key standing practices in Yi Quan. All the theories explored in this book ultimately come down to this exercise, because it signifies departing from theory and entering application.

+ Besides all the requirements for this exercise, you should never let go of the great balloon visualization, which you should adopt in this case too.

EXERCISE 8: HUN YUAN ZHUANG 浑元桩 VARIANT 2

External instructions

+ From the previous position (exercise 7), turn the palm of the back hand to face the palm of the front hand, as in the photo below.

+ The other demands are the same as in exercise 7.

Visualization

+ Imagine a balloon between your hands. Try to mentally move it forwards and backwards, up and down, and left and right with the power of your Yi-intention. The body should be completely relaxed, and the whole movement should be done with intention.

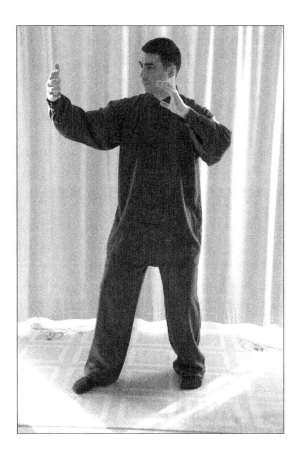

NOTES

+ Do not forget the great balloon theories. Movement in any of the six directions should encompass the idea of an existing opposing force.

+ Try to experiment with mentally moving this ball and explore the various feelings that you can obtain from this process.

+ The balloon is still moved through the power of the dan tian, and not the hands. The purpose of the hands is always to support the balloon and not to move it.

EXERCISE 9: NIAO NAN FEI ZHUANG 鸟难飞桩
External instructions

+ The requirements for this posture are the same as for hun yuan zhuang (exercise 7).

+ The hands in this case are made into loose fists as if you are holding two small birds.

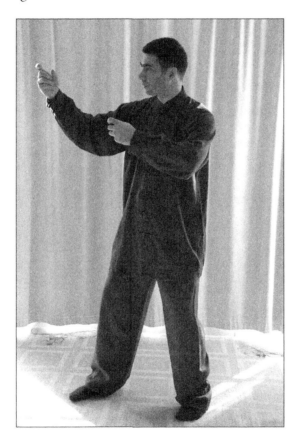

Visualization

+ The visualization for this exercise is given in the external instructions. Imagine that you are holding two birds in your hands and that they wish to fly away. However, each time they try to leave your hands, you grasp them and prevent them from escaping. The birds are not flying away from each hand at the same time, and they try to fly in random directions. You should explore as many possibilities as possible.

NOTES

- In this exercise, although the fingers slightly move, the grasping of the birds is not done with the fingers, but with the dan tian. Sometimes it helps if you imagine that there are strings attached to the feet of the birds and your dan tian. In this way, every time they try to fly away your dan tian pulls them down, and the grasping of the fingers follows.

- With this exercise you learn to coordinate the movement of your fingers with the dan tian efficiently.

CHAPTER 5

Moving the Balloon

A very important aspect of Yi Quan theory is called the "Test of Force" (shi li 试力). Understanding this type of exercise is pivotal to understanding Yi Quan. However, in medicine, it is a very important training method for both needling exercises and tui na training.

As all Chinese-speaking practitioners of Yi Quan have probably noticed, many of the names of the various "Test of Force" exercises have the word "ball" or "balloon" (qiu 球) in their name. The main point is that, in each of these exercises, you are supposed to hold an imaginary ball in your hands. Consequently, each time, you must try to figure out how your balance will affect your body coordination within the great balloon while performing the task.

The first exercise in this chapter does not appear in the Yi Quan syllabi, but it is quite common in other internal arts, such as Tai Ji Quan and Ba Gua Zhang, and is quite an important exercise in my daily personal training.

EXERCISE 10: TAI JI BALL 太极球
External instructions and visualization

✦ Assume the basic health stance; imagine being inside the great balloon.

✦ Place your hands above your belly button.

- Imagine the qi of the whole body gathering in the belly, forming a fast-spinning ball made of qi in your dan tian.

- The movement of the hands follows (but does not dictate) the spinning movement of the sphere of qi.

- The ball pops out of the belly, and between the hands.

- The movement of the ball is strictly coordinated with the movement of the belly.

- With the palms always facing one another, follow the movement of the orb. The body tries to maintain balance and harmony within the great balloon, so adapts continuously according to the movement of the sphere.

- The ball expands and the movement becomes bigger; it contracts and becomes smaller.

- Play with the ball for a few minutes at various speeds maintaining your balance, coordination and with the palms facing each other.

- The sphere becomes small again, and the movement speeds up; then you pop it back inside the dan tian, and you place your palms above the belly button.

- Take a few minutes and concentrate on the fast-spinning ball inside your belly until its qi disperses inside the body.

NOTES

- I cannot stress enough the importance of this exercise for the development of coordination between up and down, left and right, and front and back, as well as whole body balance. In my experience, this exercise is the first step towards understanding the basics of shi li. You get to feel the imaginary ball, play with it and in some cases use footwork to walk or move around it, while maintaining all the attributes of hun yuan li theory.

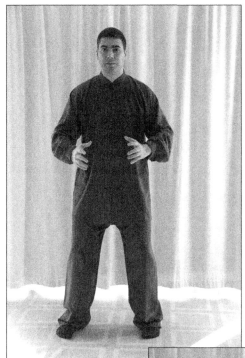

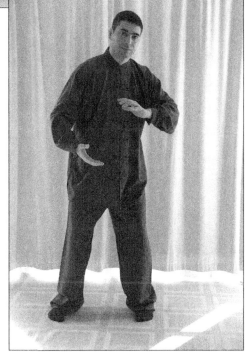

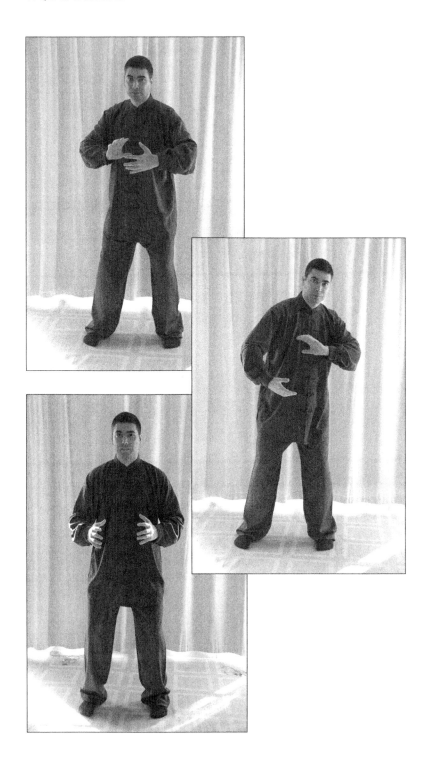

EXERCISE 11: PING TUI SHI LI 平推试力
External instructions and visualization

+ From fu an zhuang (exercise 5), imagine you are standing in the middle of a lake or the sea.

+ Your hands are resting on top of a wooden plank (or a balloon) floating at the level of the chest, with palms down.

+ With your belly, and not the power of your hands, try to push the plank forwards and then pull it backwards.

+ Feel the resistance coming from the water when you move back and front.

+ Feel the resistance coming from the plank from three directions: up, back and front.

NOTES

+ As you pull, your body sinks, and as you push, your body stands up. Breathing should be normal and independent of the movement of the plank (or balloon). There is an imaginary stick, loosely connecting your belly with the plank, so every time the plank moves it is through the power of the belly. The arms never initiate the movement, but just follow. Relaxation is very important. One of the important demands is that you should think that the movement is really big, but your body should only move slightly.

+ If you wish to do this in the ding ba bu position, when you push, your feet should go from the 70–30 position to 50–50, and then when you pull back, they should return to 70–30. You should never exceed 50–50.

+ Try to feel the resistance of the water when you move, but always mentally. Never tense your body to produce such an effect.

+ If you decide to use the balloon visualization instead of the wooden plank, your palms should adapt accordingly.

♦ You also can try to imagine that your fingers are tied on trees far away, and explore how this affects your body movement when you try to pull.

♦ Make sure that you retain balance, harmony and coordination in every movement, and that you use your whole body and not just the arms.

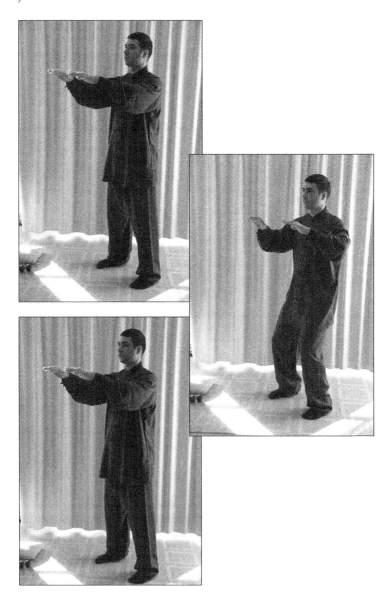

Orthodox

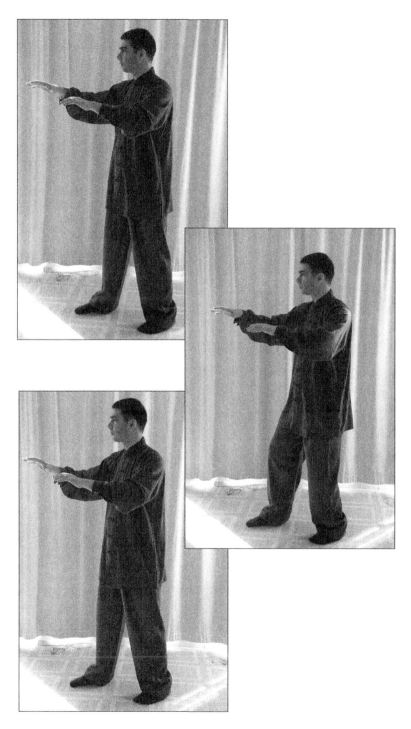

Variant

EXERCISE 12: KAI HE SHI LI 开合试力
External instructions and visualization

+ From fu an zhuang (exercise 5), turn your palms facing one another, as if holding a balloon.

+ Imagine the balloon expanding, and your body adapting to this to maintain balance and harmony.

+ As the balloon expands, you sink.

+ Then imagine the balloon shrinking, and your hands following its walls, so it doesn't fall to the ground.

+ As the balloon shrinks, you rise.

NOTES

+ If you wish to do this in the ding ba bu position, when you open (expand), your feet should go from the 70–30 position to 50–50, and then when you shrink, they should return to 70–30. You should never exceed 50–50.

+ Imagine that you are immersed in honey, and while you move, the stickiness prevents you from doing so.

+ Make sure that you maintain a good mood and quietness, that there is focus, harmony and balance in your movement, and that you explore these during the exercise.

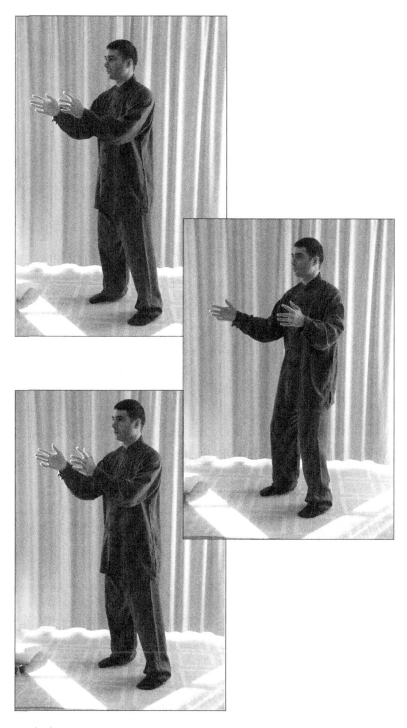

Orthodox

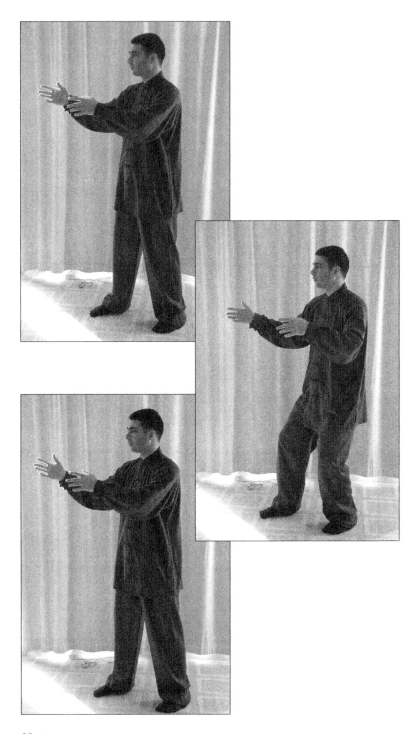

Variant

EXERCISE 13: FU AN QIU SHI LI 扶按球试力
External instructions and visualization

+ From fu an zhuang (exercise 5), imagine that the balloon is rising up to eyebrow level.

+ Follow its movement so that it doesn't escape. However, in this exercise it is the body that follows it, and the hands merely have the supporting role.

+ After the balloon reaches the level of the eyebrows, try to push it back with your whole body, until it reaches its original place.

+ The movement continues unbroken, and externally it looks almost like drawing water out of a well.

+ When the balloon rises, your whole body rises up.

+ When you pull the balloon back, you sink.

+ Imagine that you are still immersed in honey. Try to understand the contradictory forces that are involved in this exercise through meticulous research and reasoning.

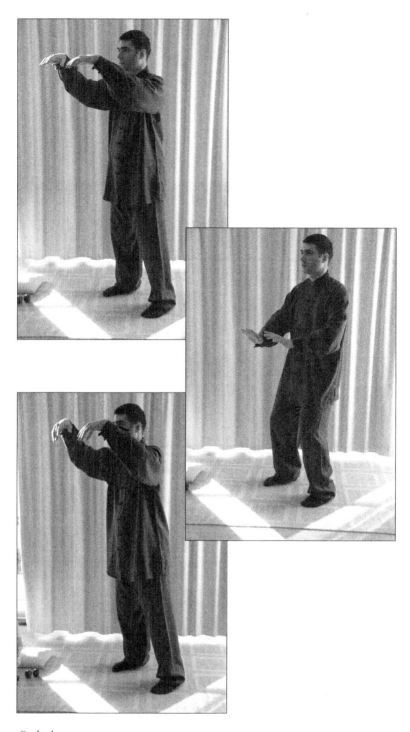

Orthodox

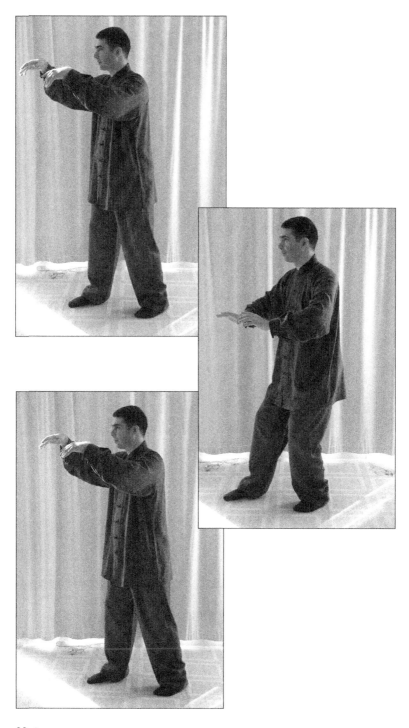

Variant

CHAPTER 6

Acupuncture and Zhan Zhuang

As promised in the Introduction, here I detail the various exercises that I developed through my journey. I hope that others will also find them useful in their clinical practice.

EXERCISE 14: HUN YUAN ZHUANG NEEDLING THROUGH THE HU KOU
External instructions

+ From the cheng bao zhuang position (exercise 3), the right (or left) foot moves forwards for a half step. The back foot turns outwards, forming an angle of approximately 45° with the front foot, and the position of the two feet roughly resembles the Chinese character ba 八. This foot positioning is referred to as the ding ba bu 丁八步 position.

+ The demands for ding ba bu are that the front foot is not too far forwards, and that there is a comfortable and natural feeling rather than rigidity.

+ The heel of the front foot is slightly raised, as if there is a sheet of paper underneath it.

+ Your weight should be distributed 30 percent on the front foot, and 70 percent on your back foot.

+ The feeling is that your buttocks are sitting comfortably on a giant balloon.

+ The hands are level with the chest.

+ Imagine that with the needling hand you are holding an acupuncture needle, which aims directly through the hu kou (the area between the thumb and the pointing finger) of the supporting hand.

+ Imagine that the supporting hand is holding a cotton ball.

+ The movement of the needle is strictly directed by the dan tian through the course of the lung channel.

+ The tip of the imaginary needle, your nose and your toe form a straight line.

+ The eyes focus on the cotton ball, and the Yi 意 projects directly towards the imaginary point of penetration.

+ The distance between the hands is still about 2–3 fists.

+ Relax the shoulders.

+ The tongue softly touches the palate.

+ The abdomen is relaxed and round, and the chest slightly drawn in.

+ You should not use any force, but all the imaginary movement should be done with the power of the Yi-intention.

NOTES

+ Relaxation, harmony and coordination are important demands for this exercise. In this zhuang you should try to project your intention towards the point of the needle.

+ Be aware of the various contradictions, and try to change rigidity into softness, and also clumsiness into proficiency.

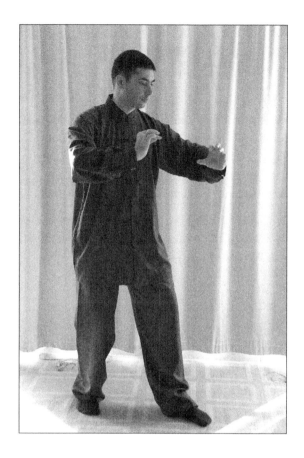

Additional visualizations

✦ Imagine that the needle is full of small hooks, which prevent it from entering or being removed. Try to mentally work out the contradictions.

✦ The needle is stuck firmly. You should use your Yi to warm and activate the muscle area around the needle so it can release it.

✦ There is no De Qi 得气 feeling. You should use your Yi to project the qi so it can activate the point.

✦ The point feels hollow and empty. You should use your Yi to seek solidity in the emptiness.

EXERCISE 15: HUN YUAN ZHUANG NEEDLING THROUGH THE PAPER STACK
External instructions

- ✦ From the cheng bao zhuang position (exercise 3), the right (or left) foot moves forwards for a half step. The back foot turns outwards, forming an angle of approximately 45° with the front foot, and the position of the two feet roughly resembles the Chinese character ba 八. This foot positioning is referred to as the ding ba bu position.

- ✦ The demands for ding ba bu are that the front foot is not too far forwards, and that there is a comfortable and natural feeling rather than rigidity.

- ✦ The heel of the front foot is slightly raised, as if there is a sheet of paper underneath it.

- ✦ Your weight should be distributed 30 percent on the front foot, and 70 percent on your back foot.

- ✦ The feeling is that your buttocks are sitting comfortably on a giant balloon.

- ✦ The hands are level with the chest.

- ✦ With the needling hand you are holding a real acupuncture needle, which is inserted with small movements into a paper stack held by the supporting hand.

- ✦ The movement of the needle is strictly directed by the dan tian through the course of the lung channel.

- ✦ As you face forwards, the tip of the needle, your nose and your toe form an imaginary straight line.

- ✦ The eyes focus on the point of penetration, and the Yi projects directly towards the tip of the needle.

- ✦ Relax the shoulders.

- ✦ The tongue softly touches the palate.

- ✦ The abdomen is relaxed and round, and the chest slightly drawn in.

+ You should not use any force, but all the entire movement should be done with the power of the Yi-intention and the force of the dan tian.

+ Needle movement should be very small to reflect the reality of needling a real patient. Avoid overly large, sudden and uncoordinated movement.

+ Be aware that, when you needle in, you are actually needling a patient and not a paper stack.

+ Try to insert the needle without bending it, in one smooth and graceful movement. (Also avoid pricking yourself.)

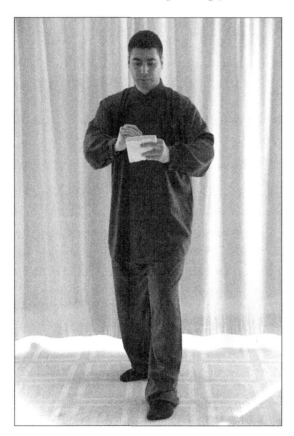

NOTES

+ The focus of this exercise is the training of the finger force and the Yi.

+ Additional visualizations from exercise 14 also apply.

EXERCISE 16: HUN YUAN ZHUANG NEEDLING THROUGH THE COTTON BALL

This exercise is basically the same as exercise 15, but in this case the visualizations and the training tool are different.

Visualizations

+ While inserting the needle in the cotton ball, you should focus on training the different hand manipulations. It is very important that you try to connect your dan tian with your needling and supporting hand, and internalize every single hand manipulation.

+ This is the same as what Master Cui Fu-shan called "internalization of external exercises."

+ Your Yi still projects towards the tip of the needle.

+ Again, perform only small manipulations, and always visualize that you are needling a real person. All of your training must have a realistic focus, otherwise it will lead to danger in practice.

Additional training tools

The above exercise can also be performed with two additional tools:

+ *Tofu:* Fresh tofu is a type of material that is both very soft and very brittle. If your lifting and thrusting is not done perpendicularly, the tofu will break apart. Exercising with pieces of tofu will teach you some needling control. (Be careful not to create a mess.)

+ *Wooden cube with hole:* This is a wooden cube with a hole in the middle. You hold it with your hand and you aim for the hole, trying to insert the needle without hitting the mouth or its walls. This exercise will help in developing your aim, especially if you enjoy needling without a guiding tube.

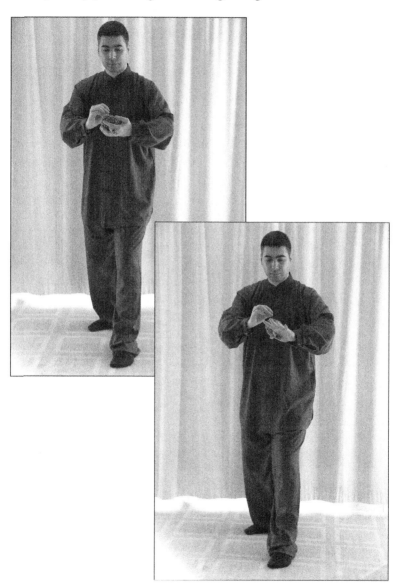

Additional shielding and cleansing exercises

I have heard from many friends practicing acupuncture that they often feel exhausted and drained after seeing only a few patients a day. In accordance with the demands of "Nourishing the Spirit," I present here two additional exercises about shielding and cleansing, in accordance with Yi Quan for health.

EXERCISE 17: HOLDING YOUR SPEAR AND SHIELD TO PROTECT YOURSELF

While needling, imagine, as in the hun yuan zhuang posture, the supporting hand holding your shield and the needling hand holding the spear (needle). Visualize the shield being made of light and fire, and no evil can go through. (Also please refer to the visualization for exercise 7.)

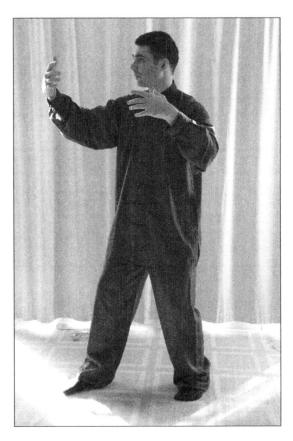

EXERCISE 18: RAIN TAKES AWAY THE DIRT

After the patient has left the treatment room, open the window for the fresh qi to enter. Do not accept another patient for a few minutes. Stand in "ti cha zhuang" (exercise 1), and imagine warm rain falling from the sky, penetrating even the deepest parts of your body and cleansing away all evils. Also imagine urinating without urinating, and through the imaginary urine all evils are driven away. All of this imaginary bad energy leaves the room, and you should visualize that it disappears or burns away. After you have regained your energy and focus, then you can welcome your next patient in. (Also please refer to exercise 1, visualization 4.)

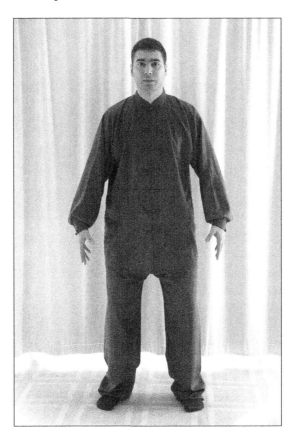

Training of the Wrist Force and Discussion on Other Needling Skills

The acupuncture needle is a very thin, wiry and flexible medical instrument. Inserting it in the body of the patient is by no means an easy feat, and acupuncturists usually spend years before they are able to effectively, accurately, steadily and safely administer acupuncture treatment.

As we have explored in the chapter about Zhi Shen (Controlling the Spirit), a correct mindset and concentration is vital before one is able to provide effective treatment. On the other hand, realistic training should also focus on the connection of the internal with the external skills 内外合一, which also include possessing the correct finger force, having good control over the depth, direction and angle of the insertion, and proficiency in the various reinforcing or reducing techniques, with the needle being an extension of the whole body.

In most of the exercises presented earlier in this book, the requirements were that both the left and the right sides of the body are trained evenly. However, in practical administration of acupuncture needling, there is a fundamental difference. Usually in the classics, the right hand is described as the "puncturing or needling hand," while the left hand is termed the "supporting or pressuring hand." However, this is not really a law, and people can adapt according to which side they feel comfortable using.

However, in my opinion, both hands are of equal importance, and according to whole body theory (imagine balancing left and right inside the great balloon) the way each one acts will certainly reflect on the outcome of the treatment.

In this book I have described how to needle through the paper stack or the cotton ball while practicing Zhan Zhuang meditation. However, for some comprehensive techniques such as "Setting the Mountain on Fire" or the "Heaven Penetrating Cooling Method," where the depth of the needling and accuracy of manipulation is of vital importance, the paper stack can be placed on a table, with the supporting hand fixing it in position and the needling hand practicing the comprehensive puncturing technique.

Besides finger force, some acupuncturists also believe that the strength and softness of the muscles around the carpal, metacarpal and phalangeal bones is quite important. Therefore wrist force is also considered an important skill to pursue, especially as it can help in transmitting the needling sensation more easily across the channels.

Here I present five traditional exercises that may assist fellow acupuncturists, and also tui na therapists, to develop this skill.

Finger meditation standing

Finger meditation standing has two variants. The first is mostly used in acupuncture for practicing wrist force; the second is used in tui na for meditating on the character an 按 (pressing).

EXERCISE 19: DOUBLE THUMB MEDITATION
Basic demands

+ Stand close to the table.

+ Imagine that you are inside the great balloon.

+ Your center of gravity is your dan tian—become aware of it.

+ Keep silent, and concentrate on your breathing.

+ Relax deeply, and sink the qi to the dan tian.

+ Extend your arms forwards with the thumbs together.

+ Bend slightly forwards, and gently place the thumbs on the edge of the table, exerting only slight pressure.

+ Do not place your weight on the thumbs—your center of gravity is still your dan tian.

+ Concentrate on the thumbs for five minutes.

+ Repeat twice a day.

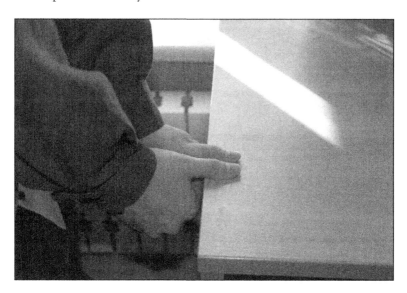

EXERCISE 20: INDEX FINGER AND THUMB MEDITATION
Basic demands

+ Stand close to a table.

+ Imagine that you are inside the great balloon.

+ Your center of gravity is your dan tian—become aware of it.

+ Keep silent, and concentrate on your breathing.

+ Relax deeply, and sink the qi to the dan tian.

+ Place a soft pillow on the table.

+ Make a hook shape with the index fingers of both hands.

+ Bend slightly forwards, and gently press the pillow with the middle phalanx of the index finger and the tip of the thumb.

+ Do not place your weight on the fingers as this may hurt— your center of gravity is still your dan tian.

+ Concentrate on the meaning of the character an, pressing for five minutes.

+ Repeat twice a day.

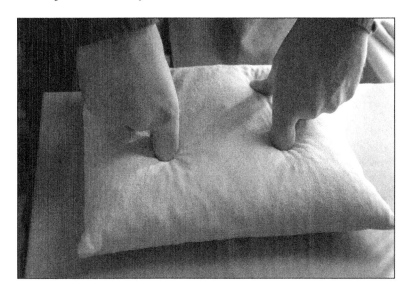

NOTES

+ Although this is not necessarily an acupuncture training method, it does help to train concentration, patience and wrist force.

EXERCISE 21: THREE FINGERS HITTING METHOD
Basic demands

+ Stand close to a table.

+ Imagine that you are inside the great balloon.

+ Your center of gravity is your dan tian—become aware of it.

+ Keep silent, and concentrate on your breathing.

+ Relax deeply, and sink the qi to the dan tian.

+ Make a hook with the index and middle fingers of the needling hand, and press their tips with the tip of the thumb.

+ Using whole body movement, hit the fingers on a book placed on the table.

+ The movement of the supporting hand dictates the movement of the needling hand. To understand this, consider the Chinese rattle drum with the two wooden balls. The movements of both sides are interdependent.

+ Repeat 100–150 times a day.

+ Hit the fingers very gently. Hitting hard will not speed up the process, and it may also hurt your hand. The demand here is to train the accuracy of the movement, and not any type of finger strength.

Other exercises
EXERCISE 22: HITTING THE BAG OF BEANS
This exercise comes from the basic training of Tong Bei Quan. The bean-bag is usually made of leather or thick cloth, and is about the size of A4 paper. It is then filled with soybeans.

External instructions

+ From the ding ba bu position, grasp the bag with the supporting hand.

+ Imagine being inside the great balloon, with your center of gravity being the dan tian.

+ Using whole body action, with the needling hand you strike the bag with your palm or your fist, performing a similar movement to kai he shi li (exercise 12).

+ When you strike the bag, the supporting hand (left), nose and the big toe of the left foot should be on the same line.

+ When you strike, the weight on the feet goes from the 70–30 position to 30–70 at the point of hitting, and then when you retreat it returns to 70–30. This is originally a fighting exercise, and therefore it allows more space for larger movement. In some cases you can do this exercise with stepping, but always make sure that the fist lands at the same time as the front foot steps forward, to maintain coordination.

+ Avoid overly large, sudden and uncoordinated movement.

+ The eyes should focus on the bag.

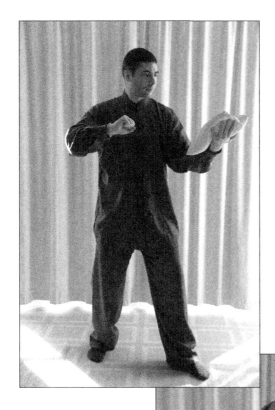

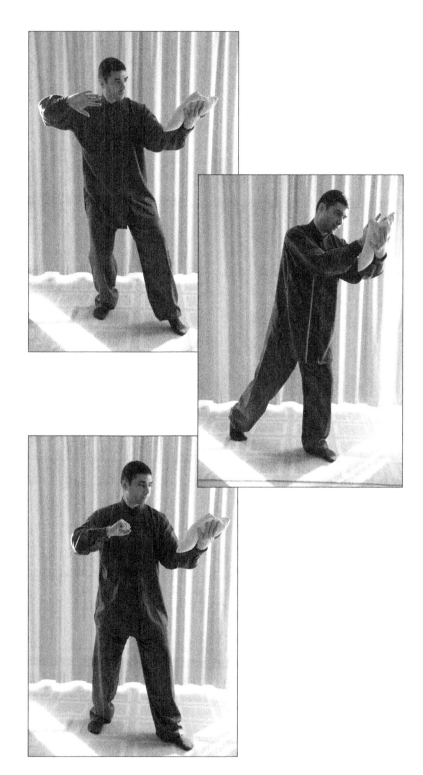

NOTES

+ The basic demands for this exercise are similar to kai he shi li (exercise 12). However, because there is hitting involved, the practitioner often feels the painful sensation associated with repeated hitting. The purpose of this exercise is to practice the soft whole body hitting (for tui na), and also relaxing the muscles of the palm and wrist for both tui na and acupuncture. When you can strike with the whole body and your palm has become soft enough not to feel any discomfort, then you have reached the necessary level. You can train in this exercise on both sides, and also for martial applications.

EXERCISE 23: HOLDING BAO DING BALLS
External instructions

+ Assume the stance of niao nan fei zhuang (exercise 9).

+ Concentrate on your breathing.

+ Sink the qi to the dan tian.

+ Instead of imagining holding the two birds, this time you hold two bao ding balls with your needling hand.

+ Try to move the balls with the power of the dan tian.

+ Imagine being inside the great balloon, and try to maintain balance in every direction throughout the course of the entire movement.

+ Do not over-do it at the beginning.

+ Try to be gentle and relaxed, and appreciate the movement of the balls as they follow the movement of the whole body.

+ Rolling the balls faster won't make this skill develop more quickly.

+ Keep doing this for as long as you can.

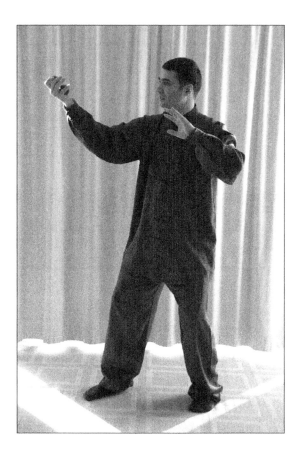

Notes

+ Avoid doing this exercise too rigidly, and try to understand how the movement of the whole body affects the movement of the bao ding balls. Softness, gentle rolling, coordination, balance and concentration will produce the correct skill.

+ In other variations of this, you can change sides, or hold sets of bao ding balls with both hands.

EXERCISE 24: TRAINING WITH THE TAI JI RULER
External instructions

+ With the hands at the extended position from ping tui shi li (exercise 11), hold the ends of the tai ji ruler with your fists.

+ Imagine yourself being inside the great balloon.

+ Sink the qi to the dan tian.

+ Become aware of your breathing.

+ With the right fist, rotate the ruler forwards, while the left slides unobstructed in the opposite direction.

+ During the movement, maintain balance and coordination between the two hands.

+ When the movement of one hand is true, the movement of the other is empty and vice versa. Work out this contradiction in your mind.

+ The entire course of movement is dictated by the dan tian.

NOTES

+ If you do this exercise too rigidly it may hurt your wrists. Imagine being on a boat that moves according to the waves, with your hands and your body following that movement. Always do each movement gracefully, softly and balanced. Avoid any stiffness and robotic movements. This exercise is very common in Bu Enfu's Yi Quan and Shuai Jiao lineage for the training of wrist strength, small movement and the coordination of right and left. (In the photos that follow, a much bigger movement is shown for demonstration purposes.)

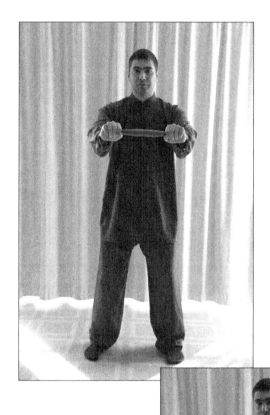

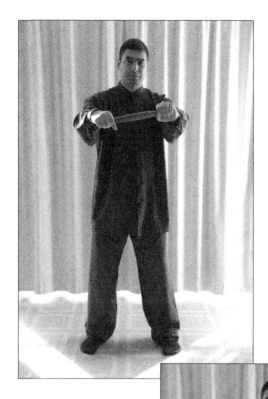

CHAPTER 8

Essentials of Zhan Zhuang Practice

Looking at the big picture, the point of Zhan Zhuang—and Yi Quan in general—is not only to assist your martial, health or spiritual awakening and cultivation but, most importantly, it helps you discover your place in the cosmos. Your body is a micro-reflection of society and the universe. If you understand how your body works, then you can—by extension—reflect further on any other problem, no matter how big or small, and discover the correct solution. This means that your body and your experiences become the yardstick by which you can judge any situation and eventually become a true master-scholar. And every time you see something being out of place, you can immediately identify it and correct it.

Wang Xiang-zhai began several of his essays with words about respecting the elders, helping the country, aiding others, being humble and hardworking, and exercising benevolence. He also spoke about being clear about what skill you wish to achieve through your training, and the reason why you wish to achieve it.

Yi Quan therefore is a small Tao, and not only a path to martial excellence and health preservation.

History will probably describe our times as the era of poison. And undeniably there is so much poison everywhere. It lingers in the water, the food, the soil, the plants and the air, and even dwells in our hearts and minds, our modern-day morality, our family values and our declining standards of education. The modern Western lifestyle is by principle very stressful. When growing up in rural Greece, I remember that every day the shops would close at about 2pm, and families would go back home and have lunch together around the table. Everybody took a short nap and, fully refreshed, went back to work at 5pm. This daily routine augmented family relationships, and everyone was able to release their stresses, laugh, discuss, share their daily adventures and carry on with their tasks in the afternoon with much newfound energy.

Later, when I moved to London, the lifestyle was different. Everything was hurried and free time was a rarity. Most jobs would be "results oriented" and performed with a "can do" attitude. There was no replenishing of energies at mid-day, and people would only meet back home in the evening, too exhausted to do anything.

Back in 2002, China was still quite a heart-warming place to live, where human interaction, understanding and friendships were true and unpretentious. However, after over a decade of continuous development, people have changed. I will not speak much about the social transformation of modern China, but it saddens me to see that people have—to a great extent—lost their smile, openness and sense of propriety. Work stress, interacting with people who carry all kinds of bad energies, bad eating habits, lack of exercise, prolonged hours of sitting or standing, breathing the polluted air of the north and inappropriate housing or dressing eventually bring up stiffness, stagnations and obstructions to the normal flow of energies within the body. These stagnations, poisons and evils linger within our body for many years and adversely affect our health.

One of the main points of the health aspect of Zhan Zhuang is the ability to allow the muscles to relax and encourage the free flow of qi and blood. This can promote health and recovery at the deepest level.

Therefore, when initially adopting any Zhan Zhuang posture, the major requirement is to derive an overall feeling of comfort, coordination and relaxation. Breathing should be natural, and the heart should not receive any extra strain such as from overwork.

A variety of visualizations used in exercises have the purpose of assisting your mind and body to become as one, by teaching control and coordination, aiding in developing the intention 意 and whole body power 浑圆力, and facilitating relaxation in every movement.

During practice one should avoid strong feelings, such as worry, sadness, stress, fear and overconfidence. Instead one should adopt a good mood and realistic expectations, and actively seek to develop a deeper understanding.

It doesn't matter if you cannot hold a posture for a very long time; everybody should practice only for as long as they feel comfortable. Eventually the practicing time will increase naturally. Any forced attempts will only negatively affect progress. However, although you should not push yourself, you should try to train meticulously and patiently.

Eventually, after becoming able to maintain the Zhan Zhuang feeling for lengthy periods of time, you will be able to train harder, and at the same time the qi and blood will flow unobstructed inside the body, efficiently nourishing the internal organs, muscles, bones and tendons. The qi in the meridians will move harmoniously and the internal and external harmonies will be able to coordinate efficiently. At that stage, if someone wishes to pursue the martial variant, exercise can become more intensive while the effort of the brain and the heart decreases. This is what Wang Xiang-zhai called "training and resting becomes as one" and also "performing demanding exercises, while not placing any extra burden on the heart."

For beginners, it takes some time to acquire this feeling, especially because over the years the body has accumulated many stresses, bad habits, qi and blood blockages which prevent the muscles relaxing, and therefore create many stagnations.

Therefore, traditionally, at the basic level, one should never train for more than 2–3 postures in one sitting. Changing from one posture to the next too early and too often will disrupt the balance of the qi and blood movement, and create more harm than benefit. However, after reaching proficiency, when all postures have become part of one's natural movement, this rule can be disregarded.

From the 意拳正轨
(The Right Path of Yi Quan)
Six Harmonies

The Six Harmonies are divided into Internal and External. It is said that: the Heart should be in harmony with the Mind (Yi), the Mind should be in harmony with the Qi, and the Qi should be in harmony with the Force (Li). These are the Three Internal Harmonies.

The Hand should be in harmony with the Foot, the Elbows should be in harmony with the Knees, and the Shoulders should be in harmony with the Waist. These are the Three External Harmonies.

Elsewhere, it has also been said: concerning the Tendons and Bones, these should be in harmony with the Muscles. The Lung should be in harmony with the Kidney. These are the Three Internal Harmonies.

The Head should be in harmony with the Hand, the Hand should be in harmony with the Body, and the Body should be in harmony with the Foot. These are the Three External Harmonies.

In general, if the Mind is in harmony, the Strength is in harmony, and if the Body Axis is in harmony, the methods of the whole body are mutually combined in harmony.

This is not about how various body parts are combined in harmony. Alas, the Six Harmonies mislead many people. People who study this should be very cautious.

Wang Xiang-zhai said that moving exercises (such as the shi li presented earlier) train the muscle and bones, while standing training (such as the various Zhan Zhuang exercises) trains the zheng qi and creates abundance of the three treasures of shen, qi and jing. Therefore, one should train in both types of exercises. It is very important that every exercise should have a purpose in order to efficiently train the intention 意 otherwise even the hardest and longest training regime will yield no fruit. Although all exercises have sets of rules, the form, visualizations and intention should always be quite flexible. This is because the practitioner should always be able to efficiently adapt in the face of changing situations.

After attaining some proficiency, you should be able to direct your intention towards achieving a certain therapeutic goal. Consistent training will assist in accumulating enough shen, qi and jing, and together with sheltering you should be able to protect yourself from invading negative energies.

The *Huang Di Nei Jing* advises as follows:

A continuous failure to induce a curative effect is due to the acupuncturist's inability to concentrate his spirit essence. When one pays no attention to the mind and intention, his internal and external [harmonies] will be in disagreement, and this will give rise to doubt and may lead to danger.

Wet towel paradigm

Master Cui Fu-shan used to say that, before administering treatment, one's hands should develop a type of "friction force" (mo ca li) according to the analogy of a wet towel.

Imagine a towel representing your hands. If it is dry, and you try to pull it across an equally dry and smooth surface, you will realize that it moves quite effortlessly. It never becomes attached to the surface, and the "energies" cannot connect.

However, if the towel is wet, dragging it across the same smooth surface won't be as easy, and it will stick to the surface, thus creating a connection. The ability to form this connection is the skill that one should seek through meditation.

If the practitioner's hands are stiff, their force is dry, much like a dry towel. The manipulations will never reach the deep level, and they will resemble poking someone with a stick. If you continue to practice in this manner, the stiffness will eventually damage your patient's muscles and ligaments and your own.

However, if the practitioner learns to relax, the qi and blood will move unobstructed and naturally produce the wet towel effect. Developing this ability will allow you to listen better to the patient's body and effectively adapt your manipulation approach. Also, your treatment will reach much deeper without creating any physical damage.

Regulating the breath, heart and form

During practice, one should be able to regulate one's breath 调息, heart 调心 and form 调形.

The regulation of the heart requires that one trains their mind to focus, standing alone in the face of the cosmos. The practitioner becomes one with the heaven and the earth. There is a natural echo between the muscles, the surrounding air, structures and the floor. There should be a feeling of agility, lightness and comfort. After practice, every movement, every breath and every thought is strongly integrated with the adjacent space. Every movement affects everything around you, and even the slightest breeze will move you.

The mood should be pleasant. The mind should be free of disturbing thoughts and empty, with the body relaxed, balanced and in harmony. There should not be any stress, need, urgency or unrelated feeling. You should practice your patience and character and be serious about what you seek to accomplish. Eventually, through this process, internal and external harmony will develop naturally.

To regulate the breath in Yi Quan, one does not need to imagine the breath descending to the dan tian as in other arts. Here the requirement is that the breath is natural, even and comfortable. The heart does not receive any extra burden from complicated breathing practices, and the flow of qi in the body remains even and naturally regulated. This can help the continuous progress and developing of one's strength without taxing the body and creating imbalances and stagnations.

Regulating the form is one of the most important stages in training. In many Chinese arts there exists the concept of the whole body force. This is an ancient concept, even appearing in the *Huang Di Nei Jing*, when it says that the ancient sages trained with all their muscles working as one 肌肉若一.

In Yi Quan we seek this force through mentally unraveling the concept of contradictions 矛盾. This entails exploring a variety of physical and spiritual qualities through deciphering their Yin and Yang dichotomies. In the physical we seek force in the six directions of up–down, left–right and front–back, and eventually reach a situation where one achieves complete control of their movement in any direction. In terms of the surrounding space, one must observe, study and adapt to the changes of the environment, ultimately becoming, as Wang Xiang-zhai said, like "a flag in the wind, or a fish in the stream."

In the spiritual we seek to adapt to emotions, cancel out negativity, and achieve complete comfort, elasticity, patience, agility of mind and character.

The *Huang Di Nei Jing* summarizes all of the above points as follows:

> The Yellow Emperor said: I hear that in the olden days there were sages able to live in accordance with the principles of the heaven and the earth, grasp the laws of the movement of the yin and yang, breathing the essential qi, standing alone, guarding the spirit, with all the muscles working as one. Hence they can live so long as to outlive the heaven and the earth, and their life never ends. This is the Tao of life. (*Su Wen—Shang Gu Tian Zhen Lun*)

Where and when to train

Choosing a place for training is very important. Especially for beginners it has to be a place without many noises, with plenty of fresh, clean air, away from pollution, dust and strong smells. You should avoid strong, cold winds and inappropriate dress for the time of the year.

Ideally it will be in a place with trees, or some running water, or by the sea. One should avoid practicing under the strong midday sun.

Closed places such as rooms where the air is stale and dirty should be avoided. Public training in rooms without windows or proper ventilation should also not be permitted. Training with people who create disturbance, make noises and bring about negative energies should also be avoided.

In Zhan Zhuang there is no such thing as an appropriate time for training. One can always assume training at any point during the day. The requirement is not quantity but quality of training, so therefore one can practice for as long or as little as one's lifestyle permits, but each time it should be done properly and with the correct mental content. Nevertheless, for methodical training, morning exercise is best, because the city air is relatively cleaner, and also the body is relaxed and energetically recharged after an appropriate length of sleep.

While some people demonstrate an ability to continuously stand for 2–3 hours in one session, I think it is better doing three to four chunks of 5–10 minutes of training, spread throughout the course of the day.

In methodical training, beginners are usually asked to stand for 30–40 minutes, followed by another half hour of seeking forces. Full martial training requires 4–5 hours of martial applications, pushing hands and real-time fighting upon the completion of these basic exercises. However, such training ideas and methods are quite beyond the scope of this book.

Failure to concentrate during training

During practice many people find it really hard to concentrate. Random thoughts come up; the mind wanders, and concentration suffers. The best way to deal with disturbing thoughts is to let go. If you try to fight such thoughts, they will always come back. However, if you let go of them, eventually they will disappear.

On the other hand, such thoughts also turn up if there is stress, sadness and other strong emotions. In such cases, you should try to relax (perhaps in the resting position), open the window, breathe a lot of fresh air, gaze into the distance, cleanse yourself of negative energies by visualizing "warm rain washing away all evils," and adjust your breathing; then you can resume the exercise for a few minutes. If the strong emotions are overwhelming, it will be better to take a long walk, calm your emotions down, and later resume Zhan Zhuang training.

Besides the above instructions, Wang Xiang-zhai also advised that you could visualize your body being like a big furnace, which has the ability to burn away all disturbing thoughts. For some people such visualization also works.

After such thoughts disappear, then you should concentrate your Yi on the demands of the exercise that you are attempting.

Various feelings during training

During standing, various feelings often appear, such as itching, yawning, pain in the muscles—especially the shoulders—trembling of the legs, and so on. These sometimes are overwhelming and can seriously affect training. Such reactions are the outcome of the unblocking of the channels, and your body trying to balance itself out. Stress, bad sleeping habits, lack of exercise, unbalanced diet, pollution, overwork and other factors have taken their toll on your body for years. Stresses, blockages and toxins have accumulated in the body. After starting Zhan Zhuang, the body starts to open up again, and such feelings are an indication of the exercises starting to take effect.

I remember that, when I first started training with my teacher, all of my old wounds would start to itch and sometimes hurt. Eventually the pain went away, and I haven't felt a similar feeling in more than ten years. In most cases, such feelings disappear after a short period of dedicated training and usually never return.

CHAPTER 9

Final Thoughts and Conclusions

Looking back over the last 12 years I have spent in China, I have tried to retrace my steps in as much detail as possible. This included going through all of my notes from several years ago, anthologizing the useful stuff, and leaving behind everything that does not represent my current way of thinking. This procedure opened a window in time, and allowed me to recall some of my early hardships in practice and at the same time reflect upon various ideas that changed as my understanding grew. Although some old thoughts were written in a very abstract way and in a hurry, their meaning allowed me to seek further spiritual depth in my current practice. These notes acted as a compass that kept me focused while working on this book.

When I was starting my path in the art of Yi Quan, and also in Contemporary Chinese Medicine, there were very few books containing adequate information on either subject. For this reason, I always kept a detailed notebook on a variety of topics, which I still continue to update every time I discover something new. Sometimes I cross things out or re-edit paragraphs even years after they were originally written. Our knowledge is something fluid that adapts and changes in accordance with how our understanding develops over time. The way this book was produced is a testament to how this process really works.

Having these thoughts, I hope that at some point in your practice you will come across the ideas that are included in these pages. They may sound completely simplistic or extremely complicated, depending on your previous training, experience and spiritual path. In any case, if you still wish to follow these exercises, I would advise that you, too, at some point during your training, write your viewpoints next to my text and attach some loose pages containing your ideas or intuitions. Allow this path to become personalized according to your way of thinking. Master Cui Fu-shan used to say, "Your best skills will come from your own thoughts." He meant that if I blindly followed his exact instructions I would eventually become a bad copy of his teachings. But if—through his teaching—I developed and practiced my own ideas, then I could be original.

I believe that if you try to follow this advice you could also under certain conditions spiritually develop your own understanding in the art of acupuncture, and both you and your patients gain a huge benefit from the healing sessions.

While writing these lines, I am sitting in a quiet room in Guangzhou. I recently moved to the south while trying to escape the thick air pollution of Beijing, although Guangzhou is only marginally better in this respect.

While it seems ridiculous to compare the current Chinese air-quality standards with those of the developed Western countries, it is still wrong to assume that the West is not as severely polluted. I often remember riding on the London Underground on a busy day, and getting a headache from the stale air, the stress and bad energies that other people unintentionally emitted. Since we cannot live up in the mountains as hermits, learning to shield ourselves is a prudent way to avoid energetic poisoning. Because many of us have to travel to work, collecting negative energies and emotions is not the best way to start off a day of providing healing. Although we do not often realize how harmful this negativity is, we should try to understand that healing starts from first maintaining a good personal energetic equilibrium. Only then can we assist others to re-discover their balance too.

In general, this book explores much about the energetic aspects of acupuncture. While most of the people who have already attained some accomplishment in the Chinese Internal Arts can directly explore and apply these ideas, those who haven't will still need personalized guidance and direct teaching before attempting any exercises.

Since with acupuncture you manipulate qi, your energies will massively influence the outcome of any treatment session. The way you pursue this will reveal much about your understanding of Energetic Ethics (Qi De 气德). I often see acupuncturists providing healing while experiencing sadness, over-excitement or anger. Their mind is not focused on the treatment, and their thoughts linger on personal troubles elsewhere. Others are driven by greed and get stressed about seeing many patients during a day so they can maximize profit. Their actions eventually become robotic, generic and soulless, while at the same time their essence gets wasted from overworking. If your patients are very important to you, and you value the energetic connections with them, then you should try to build and maintain them, as has been described in this book. Only in this way will the treatment bring light, healing and understanding to both you and your patients.

While writing these last few sentences, in my ears I kept hearing the voices of all my teachers, martial artist friends, doctors and insightful people who have taught me something worth learning. In fact, this entire volume contains the spirit of the 12 years I spent in China, without flowery words, hidden meanings and unnecessary explanations.

This book is ultimately a union of my medical training, martial philosophy, personal ideas and the voices of all those who have positively influenced my life, perceptions and principles. This is what I offer in these pages, and I hope that my experiences, and all those pieces of seemingly random information that I managed to almost methodically put together, will also help others in developing a deeper understanding of the arts.

BIBLIOGRAPHY

Articles

1. 邵素菊， 邵素霞， 李鸿章。"刺之要，治神而有效"之我见。 (Our thoughts on the dictum: "for success in needling, you must control the spirit.") 《中华中医药杂志》 2010: 2.

2. 张耀， 刘旭光。浅谈《内经》针刺治神理论在针灸临床中的应用。 (Discussion on the theory of controlling the spirit in the *Huang Di Nei Jing*, and clinical applications.) 《湖北中医药大学学报》 2012: 5 (14).

3. "赵吉平。论《素问·宝命全形论》"凡刺之真,必先治神。 ("On adjusting energy before acupuncture" from *Su Wen*: *Bao Ming Quan Xing Lun*.) 《北京中医药大学学报》 2009: 2 (32).

4. 张树剑 赵京生。古代"神"的观念与《内经》"神"相关概念的关系探讨。 (The ancient concept of Shen, and the Shen in the *Huang Di Nei Jing* and other related concepts.) 《中国中医基础医学杂志》 2010: 3.

5. 镐; 田辉。从形神关系看"针刺治神"。 (Examination of controlling the spirit in needling through the relationship of physical form and spirit.) 《辽宁中医杂志》 2009: 4.

6. 金建丰。感悟"粗守形,上守神"。 (Insights on: "the crude maintains the frame, the superior maintains the spirit.") 《浙江中医杂志》 2010: 8 (45).

7. 徐珊宁，徐芸。浅谈治神与用针宜静。 (Discussion on controlling the spirit and appropriate meditation in needling.) 《福建中医药》 2006: 5 (37).

8. 赵百孝。略谈针刺治神中的气功因素。 (Brief discussion on the Qi Gong elements of controlling the spirit in needling.) 《陕西中医函授》 1989: 3.

9. 王文远。"凡刺之真,必先治神"是针刺的核心。 (The dictum "for all kinds of needling, you should first control the spirit" being the core of acupuncture needling.) 《中国针灸》 2009: 2.

10. 王启才。论针灸疗法的治神与守气。 (Discussion on controlling the spirit and maintaining the qi in acupuncture treatment.) 《陕西中医学院学报》 1989: 4.

11. 胥荣东，张军伟，付天昊，彭鑫。针刺治神与导引行气。 (Acupuncture with Zhi Shen and Dao Yin Xing Qi.) 《针灸临床杂志》 2007: 2 (23).

12. 杜旭，刘海燕。针刺治神守神与施术环境。 (Controlling the Spirit and Maintaining the Spirit and the treatment room environment.) 《上海中医药杂志》 2012: 1.

13. 马元。针刺治神心悟。 (Thinking of acupuncture treatment of vitality.) 《山东中医杂志》 2002: 1 (21).

14. 侯慎夫。意气功。 (Yi Qi Gong.) 《浙江中医杂志》 1958: 5 (18).

Medical books

15. （清）陈梦雷等编. 集注《古今图书集成医部全录—黄帝灵枢经/难经》。 (Complete Library of Ancient and Modern Medical Works—*Huang Di Ling Shu Jing* and *Nan Jing*.) 人民卫生出版社。北京 1959.

16. （清）陈梦雷等编。集注《古今图书集成医部全录—黄帝素问》。 (Complete Library of Ancient and Modern Medical Works—*Huang Di Su Wen*.) 人民卫生出版社。北京 1959.

17. （明）朱棣。《普济方 — 第十册 — 针灸》。 (Prescriptions for Universal Relief—Volume 10—Acupuncture.) 人民卫生出版社。北京 1959.

18. （明）杨继洲。《大字五彩针灸大成》。(The Great Compendium of Acupuncture.) 上海春明书店印行 (Republic of China print 1911–1949, exact date unknown).

19. 周子干《慎斋遗书》江苏科学技术出版社。 1987.

Yi Quan books

20. 王芗斋。《拳学宗师王芗斋文集》。 (Anthology of the Works of Martial Arts Master Wang Xiang-zhai.) 中国广播电视出版社出版。北京 2010.

21. 姚宗勋。意拳养生。(Yi Quan Health Preservation.) 北京中意武馆。北京 1988.

Purple Cloud Master's Essential Methods for Painless Needle Insertion

Published by the China Acupuncture and Moxibustion Research Society

紫雲上人述 非賣品

運鍼不痛心法

中國鍼灸學研究社印行

Foreword

Eighteenth Spring of the Republic [of China] (1929). Hanging Pot[1] on the Gate of Wu.[2] In my spare time I enjoy strolling in the old book market on Hu Long Street,[3] searching for and reading old books. It was due to [this pastime that I came across] a handwritten copy of the *Essential Methods for Painless Needle Insertion*. [The manuscript was] only a few pages long and already extremely old and worn out, [but] I really enjoyed reading it. Although the words

---

1   Hanging Pot (or bottle gourd). A popular Chinese legend says that during the time of the great plagues, in a city in Henan, an old man appeared, selling medicines on the street. Although he was not much to look at, people seemed to trust him, and each time they approached him to buy medicine he would reach inside a bottle gourd, find a small medicinal bolus, and ask them to dissolve it in water and drink. One by one, all of the people who sought his assistance were cured completely. At the end of the day, the people left the market and went back to their homes. After everybody was gone, a person called Fei Zhang-fang 费长房 saw the old man entering the bottle gourd. Realizing that this was not an easy feat, the next day he bought some meat prepared in wine and approached the old man, asking him to teach him this skill. The old man agreed, and he took him along inside the bottle gourd. Fei Zhang-fang followed the old person, learning the Tao, for ten days. After that, he returned to the outside world. Arriving back home, his family was amazed to see him alive, because he had been missing not for ten days, but for ten years. Since that time, and with the skills he had acquired, Master Fei was able to cure all illnesses, even if the patient was on the brink of death. To commemorate this legend, all ancient doctors used to hang a bottle gourd at the door of their clinics, to show that they have also entered the gate of medicine (and Tao) and can perform similar healing miracles. However, this practice has been discontinued, and probably was already rare even when this book was printed, almost a century ago. However, the expression still survives as a proverb: "悬壶济世" (xuán hú jì shì), meaning "practice medicine (hanging a bottle gourd) in order to heal all the people."

2   The Gate of Wu. Wu was an ancient kingdom covering part of the areas of modern Shanghai, Anhui, Zhejiang and Jiangsu. The expression "Hanging Pot on the Gate of Wu" points to the Classical Chinese Medicine school of thought that developed in this area of China.

3   A popular street with antique bookshops in Suzhou.

民十八年春。懸壺吳門。暇則喜涉足護龍街舊書肆中。翻檢舊籍。因得運鍼不痛心法鈔本一册。寥寥數頁。已破舊不堪。喜而閱之。文雖不工。而其法則頗切於用。述者爲紫雲上人。記者爲蘭溪金仲才氏。二氏固無從考據。然必爲百年前人而精於鍼術者。因其法則○有俾鍼醫。遂購而得之。竊思中國鍼灸學術之不振。施術者之不能避免刺痛。亦爲原因之一。因災藜棗。供諸研究鍼術者之採用焉

澹盦誌

were not elegantly edited, its method was clear-cut and practical. It was [originally] attributed to Zi Yun Shang Ren, scribed by scholar Jin Zhong-cai from Lanxi.[4] [Sadly] there is no way to confirm with certainty [anything about] these two scholars. However, they must have been experts with an excellent needling skill of centuries past. Because of its method of medical needling I purchased it. Considering that Chinese Acupuncture Art has been stagnant, and that acupuncturists can truly benefit from the painless needling skill, I have given this [manuscript] to all those who research acupuncture needling so that after the [years of] hardships the skill can flourish once again.[5]

Dan An-zhi[6]

---

4   A city in Zhejiang province.

5   The manuscript offers an odd expression about changing "pigweed into date," probably meaning to develop an average skill into a remarkable practice.

6   This is Professor Cheng Dan-an (1899–1957).

PREFACE

Acupuncture can treat the disease, and its efficacy is better than that of the herbal decoctions. Having been content with the inner gate teaching I have received under the guidance of Master Huang from Wan (i.e. Anhui), [through] the secrets of the channels and acupoints, I was able to see a part of the whole picture. The golden needle can affect nine out of ten patients. However, it is a pity that inserting the needle into the muscle through the skin is not without pain. In the second month of spring in the Gui Hai[1] year, I came to [appreciate the] fragrance [of the peach flowers] at the Xuan Dou Guan[2] [temple] at Qian Tang,[3] where I also met Zi Yun Shang Ren (Purple Cloud Master). The Master had a silver beard and his hair was like snow. His spirit was healthy and vigorous, and he was an expert in the art of needling, but not easy to [be persuaded to] treat people. We talked and discussed a lot until late at night, hoping that the Master could teach me. He dictated to me his teaching on the "Essential Methods for Painless Needle Insertion," and allowed me to take notes and pass them on to others. Upon my return [at home] and within one month [of practice] I could see results. Within 100 days I was quite proficient in inserting the needle painlessly and with ease. It is a pity that [after these events] I did not have a chance to thank the Purple Cloud Master for ten years, [so I decided] to go back to visit him the following year and pay my respects. But unfortunately the Master had passed away at the end of the spring of that year. Alas! [Zi Yun Shang Ren] had given me his essential methods only over an overnight discussion. That really was a—so-called—streak of Buddhist Karma.

---

1   The Gui Hai year repeats every 60 years. Without the emperor's name, there is no way to confirm which year it points to, so it may have been 1803, 1743 or perhaps even earlier.

2   The Xuan Dou Guan temple is famous for its more than 1000 pear trees. Liu Yu-xi (772–842) and Bai Ju-yi (772–846) both wrote poems about it.

3   In Hangzhou.

敍

鍼灸治病。效逾湯藥。自得皖門黃師一峯夫子之指示。經穴祕奧。得窺一二。金鍼所至。十可全九。惟是刺肌破膚。不免痛楚。引爲憾事。癸亥仲春。進香錢塘玄都觀。得識紫雲上人。上人銀鬚雪髮。精神矍鑠。善鍼術。而不輕爲人治。夜闌剪燭傾談。蒙上人以爲可敎。將其運鍼不痛心法。口述授予。囑記而傳之世。歸而習之。一月而效見。百日而功成。運鍼自如。絕無痛楚。十年憾事。於焉以酬。翌年往拜。已於春末圓寂矣。噫。一夕之談。遠以心法相授。豈佛說之所謂因緣也耶。抑上人其亦預知將離東

The Master knew that he would soon leave this world, and that he must seek a disciple to pass his "Essential Methods" to, so that the skill would survive and not become lost. Since [I have been entrusted with this knowledge] at the end of his life, how can I keep it a secret and not make a record [so others can benefit from it]?

Mid-autumn of the Jia Zi[4] year
Recounted by Jin Zhong-cai from Lanxi

---

4   The Jia Zi year repeats every 60 years. It could have been 1864, 1804, 1744, etc. It appears that this text was written in the author's old age, and 61 years after he met Zi Yun Shang Ren.

土巫欲以其心法而遺於塵世耶。既受上人囑。安可祕不爲

之記

甲子仲秋　　　　　　　　　蘭溪金仲才叙

Cultivating the Qi

Zi Yun Shang Ren said: Inserting the needle without [causing] pain strongly depends on the cultivation of qi. If the cultivation of qi is insufficient, its effect will be inadequate. The Tao of cultivating the qi demands waking up at the Yin hour (3–5am), sitting on a futon, feet coiled together, the two hands resting on the lap, the waist straight, the chest erect, the mouth closed, the eyes relaxed. As in meditation, [one should practice] without thinking and without worrying. The mind [should focus] on the number of breaths, [counting] from one to one hundred repeatedly and uninterruptedly. Continue until the Mao hour (5–7am). Shake your clothes before the beginning and at the end of practice. Accumulate [the qi] continuously, day by day without pause. [When the] qi is sufficient, the spirit will flourish. One hundred evils cannot invade.

Cheng Dan-an's comments: This is a Buddhist tranquil sitting [meditation] exercise. "Tranquil sitting" is the best method to cultivate the qi. One inhalation and one exhalation is one breath [cycle]. Counting the breaths is counting the qi that is inhaled and exhaled. Also the thought (i.e. mental component) should be consistent (i.e. focusing on the same principle each time). The heart and the spirit should become as one. Sitting meditation does not necessarily require sitting on a futon. It also does not necessarily demand coiling the feet. And it does not request practicing at the Yin hour. You can still practice early in the morning or late in the evening, [as long as you are] in a quiet place, away from noisy grounds, [while sitting] on a bed or a chair. But one should avoid the wind or sitting in a draft. The waist [should be] straight, the chest erect.

第一章　養氣

紫雲上人曰。運鍼不痛。端賴養氣。氣養不足。其功不著
。養氣之道。寅時起身。端坐蒲團。兩足盤起。手按膝上
。腰直胸挺。口閉目垂。一如入定。無思無慮。一心數息
。自一至百。反復無間。行之卯時。振衣始已。積日累月
。不息不間。氣足神旺。百邪不侵。

『註』此為佛家靜坐法。靜坐最能養氣。一呼一吸。是為一息。數
息者數呼吸之氣。使意念一致。心神合一也。靜坐不必拘於蒲團
，亦不必一定盤膝。亦不必一定在寅時。清晨晚間。於寂靜之處
。無呼喧之地。鋪位椅櫈。皆可行之。惟須迴避迎面之風。腰直

133

The mouth [should be] closed, the eyes relaxed, and counting the breaths. These demands should all be observed. The straightening of the waist and the erect chest ensure the [correct] upright posture. The chest opens up, the abdomen becomes full. The eyes [are] relaxed, observing inside. This way, the exterior stimuli will not confuse the heart. The mouth should be closed to prevent the cold qi from invading. Breathe in with the nose, and breathe out with the mouth, gently and relaxed. The slower the breathing, the better. Through the counting [of the breaths] the heart and the spirit become as one. With lengthy practice, the abdomen will fill with true [qi], the power of the qi will double, and the evils will not be able to invade.

胸挺。口閉目垂數息。三者不可缺一。腰直胸挺則身端正，肺張
腹滿。目垂內視，則外物不亂其心。口閉不張。則冷氣不侵。吸
之以鼻。呼之以口。宜徐宜緩。愈緩愈妙。以數計之。心神合一
。久久行之。腹部充實。氣力倍增。邪無從侵矣

三

Training of the Fingers

Zi Yun Shang Ren said: Besides cultivating the qi, one must also train the finger [strength]. The most important [factor] in inserting the needle painlessly is the strength of the fingers. Use a book, and hang it up, suspended on the wall. While doing the "tranquil sitting" [exercise] move the qi to insert the needle. The heart (i.e. intention) is concentrating on the needle. The eyes focus on the paper. Each day you should insert the needle one thousand times. After lengthy and persistent practice, the finger strength will be full and then you can use it.

Cheng Dan-an's comments: Painless needling pays much attention to the finger force. People with extraordinary skills pay much attention to the fingers. Force (strength) and also qi can bestow one [with the ability to control] metal and stone. However, if the qi is not trained enough, the finger force will also be insufficient. If the qi is full, it can transform to force. Therefore, one must first cultivate the qi, and then practice the finger [force]. Practicing both for a long time will certainly help to develop this skill. Zi Yun Shang Ren used paper [suspended] from the wall, something that is frustrating. After 2–3 months of training and [through adopting] several adjustments, [I derived] the following exercise which is relatively easier. Take a 2-inch-thick square wooden plank, and fashion a square frame [on top].

第二章　練指

紫雲上人曰。養氣之外。又須練指。運鍼不痛。指力最重。練指之法。用紙簿一。懸掛壁間。靜坐片時。運氣於指。持鍼刺之。心注於針。目射於紙。日刺千下。久行不輟。指力充實。可以用矣。

『註』運針不痛。在乎指力。試觀奇人異士。手指所注。金石爲穿力也。亦氣也。然氣不充實。則指力亦不足。氣充者。則易爲力。故先養其氣。後練其指。二者互習。積久彌彰。紫雲上人用紙簿懸於壁間行之。尙有窒礙。愚經二三月之練習。經數次之變更。以下述之法練習爲較易。以二寸方厚之木條。裝成一方架。

The size should be enough to fit a page of coarse paper (coarse toilet paper). In the four corners put 4-inch-long nails. On top, tack three or four pieces of paper. Hang it up on the wall to a height of the shoulder; the wood should be facing the wall, and the paper facing towards the outside. The two fingers, with twisting action, stick the needle fast [on the paper]. Practice back and forth. The fingers should not use force. When you can insert the needle [effortlessly] with one puncture, add 1–2 more pages. If you train for a long time, progressively adding paper [until getting up] to 1-inch thick, and if you can insert the needle effortlessly, twisting it [in one movement], then the finger force has developed enough, and you will be ready to help others.

其大小適合一粗紙（大便拭污之粗紙）四角插入四寸長尖釘。即以

粗紙繃上三四張。懸掛壁間。高與眉齊。木架憑壁。紙面向外。

即用右手拇食二指。持鍼剌入之。剌入之時。以鍼尖點於紙面。

二指捻動。疾行剌入。往返鍊習。覺手指毋須用力。即可一剌而

入。再加一二紙。久久行之，依次遞加。滿一寸厚。而能不須用

力捻入者。指力功候已到，可以出而問世矣

Handling the Needle

Zi Yun Shang Ren said: If you wish to succeed in this skill, you must have a sharp instrument. If the qi cultivation is sufficient, the finger force adequate, but the needle is blunt, it will not be of any assistance. The needle must be rounded and whole. [It must be] shiny, smooth and sleek. The top is thick, the shaft is thin, and the tip is sharp. You should sharpen [the needle] and boil it in medicine. Do not allow this [inconvenience] to irritate you; this is a skill of superior practitioners.[1]

Cheng Dan-an's comments: The advanced preparations include sharpening of your tools. [Because you are] using the needle to treat the people [you] should be very careful when selecting the needle wire. [A] damaged, very thin and uneven [needle], with the tip being blunt or hair-like, will cause much pain. In addition, the breaking of the needle is dangerous, and therefore one should be careful in selecting [it]. Thin or thick, the body of the needle should be relatively uniform, and the tip of the needle sharp. The body of the needle should be rounded and whole. [It should] not [be] rusty, nor bent or flexed. After careful selection, you should always prepare the needle through boiling [with medicine]. Then rub [it] with coarse paper a few times every day. When it becomes rounded, smooth, sleek and sharp, you can use it.

---

1   Today, safety laws and regulations dictate that all acupuncturists should handle the needles according to the information provided in the latest edition of the *Clean Needle Technique Manual for Acupuncturists: Guidelines and Standards for the Clean and Safe Clinical Practice of Acupuncture* as published by the National Acupuncture Foundation.

第三章　理鍼

紫雲上人曰。欲善其事。必利其器。氣養已足。指力已充
。鍼不銳利。無補於功。鍼須圓渾。光滑而潤。由粗而細
。其端銳利。摩之擦之。藥之薰之。不厭其煩。斯爲上乘
。

『註』工欲善其事。必先利其器。用鍼療疾。鍼絲不可不愼擇。鍼
有損傷。粗細不勻。尖鈍或毛。不僅令人劇痛。復有折斷之可虞
。故擇鍼宜愼。粗細相勻。鍼鋒銳利。鍼身圓渾。無銹蝕。不灣屈
。選擇已過。再以薰鍼法製之。日用粗紙摩擦數次。則圓潤滑利
。用之應手矣

Hand Manipulations

Zi Yun Shang Ren said:[1] The knife cuts, the needle punctures. Everyone knows pain. When the sick request needle treatment they already have the fear [of pain] in their heart. First the doctor must explain to them [about the procedure], and help them to calm and relax. Rub and pinch the acupoints to cause numbness (insensitivity). The hand should be like grabbing a tiger, the demeanor should be like holding a dragon. Use the needle tip to puncture fast into the acupoint, until reaching the correct depth. Slightly pause, twist and adjust. The method of the painless needle insertion has been attained.

Cheng Dan-an's comments: The knife cuts, the needle punctures. All people know the feeling of pain. When the patient requests acupuncture treatment, they do this as a measure of last resort. The puncturing of the needle is not really painful, but in the patient's mind there is always the fear of pain. This is an illusion [of discomfort] created by the mind. The first impression is the strongest, and dictates the [future] behavior [of the patient. Often,] if there is no pain, [the mind] makes it painful; if there is pain, it makes it even more painful. Therefore, when administering acupuncture, explain that there is no pain, in order to calm the patient's mind. Use the nail to rub, pinch and numb the [patient's] skin. And then with the sharp end of the needle and the refined force of the finger, insert the needle to the appropriate depth and stop. Stop the needle and don't move it.

---

1   Although not stated by name, this chapter focuses on some of the basic demands for Zhi Shen—"Controlling the Spirit."

第四章　手法

紫雲上人曰。刀割鍼刺。人皆知痛。病者臨鍼。已存畏心

○先爲解釋。以安其驚。揉掐其穴。使其麻木。手若握虎

○勢如擒龍。以鍼點穴。疾刺而入。至其分寸。稍停捻撥

○不痛鍼法。能事已畢

『註』刀割鍼刺。夫人皆知痛楚。病者求鍼。實出不得已。針本不甚痛。而病者心中總存痛念。幻由心造。先入爲主。已有明訓。不痛似痛。痛則更痛。故於臨針之時。解釋無痛。以安其心。於應針之穴。用爪甲揉掐。使皮膚麻木。然後藉針之銳利。指之鍊力。一刺而入達應入之分寸而止。停針不動。病者絕不覺痛。乃

If the patient doesn't feel pain then you can start manipulation, and either apply tonification or the draining method. If the patient only feels numbness and a needling sensation, but no pain, then the doctor has accomplished his mission.

漸行捻撥之法。運補瀉之功。祇覺痠楚。不知有痛。醫者之能事

畢矣

145

POSTSCRIPT

The brain dictates all of one's actions and behaviors, pain and pleasure. It also commands the [perceptions of the] colors, voice, smell, taste and touch.[1] The nervous system is divided into the central nervous system and the peripheral nervous system. In addition, [the peripheral nervous system is further] divided into the vegetative nervous system (i.e. the autonomic nervous system) and the somatic nervous system (i.e. the voluntary nervous system). Here we focus on the theme of "pain." [When] one has been cut and punctured on the skin, and he has experienced pain, this sensation is induced by the compression of the nerves. The pain nerves[2] originate at the cerebral cortex, and are distributed through the spinal cord to the whole body in the space between the muscles and the bones under the skin, as well as the internal organs. The painful sensation [can be felt the] strongest in the distal nerve endings,[3] [and] these distal nerve endings are scattered within the skin.

Therefore, needling through the skin can be abnormally painful. [But when you prick] slightly deeper [than skin level], the pain becomes less intense or even disappears. This is an observable effect. Although there is a very wide distribution of pain nerves [all over the surface of the body] some parts have more, others have less.

---

1   In the Chinese text, the following two sentences are given in reverse order. I have edited and rearranged them for accuracy in a Western medicine context.

2   The pain nerves mentioned here most likely refer to sensory nerves or sensory neurons. In my translation I have left the reference to pain nerves, as in the original Chinese text.

3   The distal nerve endings mentioned here most likely refer to the nociceptors (otherwise known as pain receptors). They are the sensory nerve endings of the sensory neurons that are usually associated with feelings of pain.

運鍼不痛心法書後

吾人一切行動舉止。痛感。快感。皆由腦神經爲之主宰。即色。聲。香。味。觸。亦無不由腦神經之主司。考神經分動物性神經。植物性神經二種。又分爲中樞部與末稍部。今就知痛之範圍而言之。吾人以物切刺皮膚而覺痛者。皆痛神經受壓之所致也。痛神經之發源，在大腦之皮質。經延髓脊髓而分佈於全身之皮下筋骨間。以及內臟。其感痛力最強者。厥爲痛神經之末稍部。神經之末稍。皆散佈於皮膚間，故針刺皮膚。其痛異常。稍深則痛減輕。甚至不痛。此其明徵。又痛神經之散佈有多寡。手足指舌唇部。較全身特多。其感觸力亦最強。背部較腹爲少。臀部腿部則更少。大概筋肉豐厚之處。痛神經之散佈爲少。感痛力亦弱。故針刺指部。其痛劇烈。刺背部則不甚覺痛也。雖然痛固在於神經。而於心靈亦有關係。武

For example, the fingers, the toes, the tongue and the lips have more in comparison to the rest of the body, and therefore are the most sensitive to the feeling of pain. The back has fewer pain nerves than the abdomen, and the hips and the legs have even fewer. Generally, in areas with large tendons and muscles, there is a smaller distribution of nerves, and [thus] the painful sensation is also less profound. [If you] needle the fingers, the pain will be severe, but [if you] prick the back, it will be less distressing.

Although the painful sensation is innately due to the nerves, it also has a strong relationship with the patient's mind. When the Saint of War (i.e. Guan Yu) was poisoned and was receiving scraping bone treatment, he was playing chess to distract himself. Then, although he was receiving surgery, he felt no pain. I have also personally had similar experiences and I can [confirm] this fact. [There was a case when] I cut my fingers with a knife, without realizing it. However, after I saw what happened, there was distress and pain. If one pays attention to what is happening, then there is pain, but if he speaks or plays chess or gambles with others, the mind forgets the pain because it is distracted [with other things]. Therefore, paying attention or ignoring [the cutting] has a great relationship with our perception of pain.

Also, the perception of pain is related to the speed of pricking and cutting. If the cutting is fast there will be little pain, because [the speed] covers the reflex, through the sudden attack on the nerve, and therefore the sensation is not immediately felt. If the needle is blunt and the hand slow, the nerves will feel the pricking effect, and will immediately emit a sensation of pain. Zi Yun Shang Ren's *Essential Methods for Painless Needling* was [developed] for reducing the painful sensation through distracting the mind to other focuses.

聖之括骨療毒。其心靈專注於棋之佈局下子。故任割而不痛。卽以吾人之親歷而言之。手指每爲利刃所破而不自知。及發覺後。始覺隱然作痛。心靈未注意也。身有痛楚。而與人暢談或奕棋賭博。竟能忘其所苦。心靈移注他處也。足見心靈之專注與不專注與痛有絕大之關係。再刺切之遲速。亦有深切之關係。刺切迅速。不甚感痛。蓋痛神經猝受襲擊。其反射性不及卽行發生。若器鈍手運。痛神經感到擊刺。卽起反射作用而劇烈疼痛矣。紫雲上人之運針不痛心法。卽移減其心靈之專注。及運用其迅速之手腕。與利用器械之精良。基心理物理哲理三者而彙成其功能也。甚願研究針灸學術而施行治療者。均手此一編而依法練習之也。不特減少病家之避免。而發揚中國鍼灸學術。實利賴焉

中華民國二十年春澹盦書於中國鍼灸學研究社

149

When the speed of the wrist is quick and the needle is superior, through the [actions of] psychology, physics and philosophy, painless needling can be achieved. Those who are very willing to research about the art of acupuncture in order to treat the sick [should] have this book at hand as the guide to practice this skill. Although it is not especially aimed at reducing the amount of sick people, it can be a good [tool] for the transmission of the art of Chinese acupuncture.

Spring of the 20th year of the Republic of China (1931)
Book by [Cheng] Dan-an for the China Acupuncture
and Moxibustion Research Society

民國二十年三月初版

版權所有 翻印必究

述者　　紫雲上人

出版兼　蘇州望亭
發行　　中國鍼灸學研究社

印刷者　蘇州西中市
　　　　文新印刷公司

Detailed Exposition of the Intention and Qi Exercise

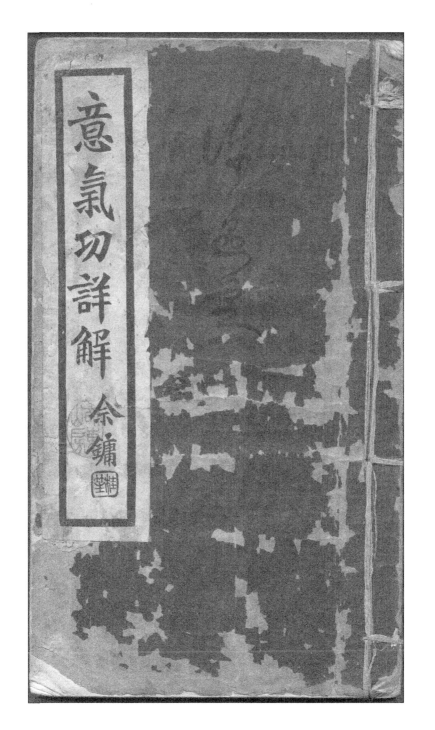

意氣切詳解　佘鏞

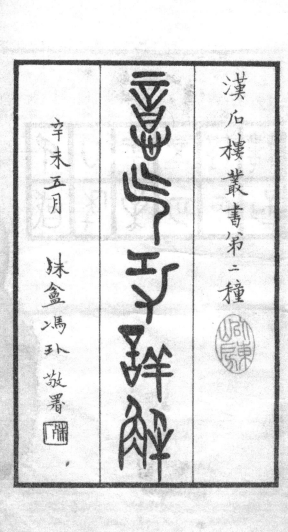

漢石樓叢書第二種

辛未五月

殊盦馮玨敬署

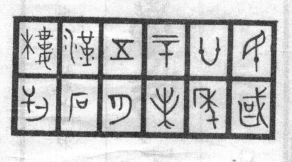

PREFACE

I lost my mother when I was eight years old. [After this event, eventually] my body became weak and frail in health, like a mere skeleton. During the Ji Si Year (1869) of Emperor Tong Zhi's 14 years of reign, the weakness prevailed. I was eating and drinking less and less every day. My father was really worried, and although I tried many therapies none of them was effective. [However,] that year I had a lucky encounter with Mr. Feng Peng-ju, a friend of teacher Ding Lan-zhai. [Mr. Feng] was 83 years old, and his spirit was healthy and strong. He understood the essence of the conversations between Qi Bo and the Yellow Emperor and the benefits of the "Intention and Qi Exercise." After he saw me he took pity and he made a direct diagnosis that I suffered from tuberculosis, which cannot be treated. He also said that this disease [manifests because] my pre-heaven essence is insufficient, and my post-heaven essence is in such a disharmony that no medicine or stone needle can provide a cure. Teacher Ding begged him again and again for a miraculous formula, but Mr. Feng said that there is no cure, except perhaps for the practice of the "Intention and Qi Exercise." [He claimed that] if I kept practicing, [eventually] the disease would become stable or even be healed. Then he personally instructed me in this exercise. [He said that] it should be practiced for 100 days without stopping. I did as instructed for the full length of that period. Then my sickly body rapidly turned to the better. Later [I continued and] it became my daily workout.

Over the last 60 years I have practiced continuously, and now I am 76 years old, in full health and my spirit essence is strong and secure. Nobody believes that during childhood I suffered from tuberculosis. I am thankful to Mr. Feng's medical ethics, who at the same time taught me the importance of physical training. Over several decades I have instructed more than 1000 relatives and friends.

自序

愚八歲失恃體質羸弱骨瘦如柴同治己巳年十四尫羸特甚飲食
日減先君憂之百計治療不見效果適遇業師丁朗齋先生之友焉
鵬舉君時年八十有三精神矍鑠精岐黃而兼善意氣功見而憐之
親加診視斷爲童子癆將不治並謂凡患此病者皆由先天不足後
天失調所致非藥石所能奏效丁師一再商請拯救之方焉先生云
無已惟有修習意氣功之一法如能持之有恒或可挽回遂面授此
功諄屬屬日內不可間斷愚如法行之及期其病體竟霍然而愈爾
後定爲日課六十年來未嘗少間今賤齒已七十有六矣頑軀健全
精神強固無論何人絕不信愚於幼時曾患童子癆者愚感焉先生
傳授之德兼提倡體育之意數十年中口授戚友不下數十百人。

159

The diseased have been cured, the weak have become strong and the healthy have turned stronger.

There were several letters[1] offering me thanks for the remarkable and impressive effects of this exercise. Therefore in order to facilitate its propagation, and explain the method of its cultivation as well as how to accomplish its effects, I have written this book and printed it to make it public for all people, and I am sure that Mr. Feng from the heavens would also be very happy for it. The true origin of this exercise is described over the next pages.

20th year of the Republic of China (1931),
Xin Wei year, first month of spring
Introduction by scholar Wang Xian-bing
(Wang Zhu-lin) from Tianjin

---

1   The beginning of this manuscript originally contained several such letters and introductions by people who used this exercise. Because they were mere endorsements, offering no real knowledge or insight, I do not include them in this edition. Various reprints of the book also do not contain them.

病者愈弱者健健者益形堅强矣書函稱謝盈篇纍牘其功效謂非

斐然可觀者乎茲爲便於傳播計將其修養之法及其功效筆之於

書付諸梓人公諸同好斯固不僅意氣功普及之幸抑亦馮先生所

含笑於地下而首肯者也際茲出版述其緣起如右

民國二十年歲次辛未孟春天津王賢賓竹林氏序

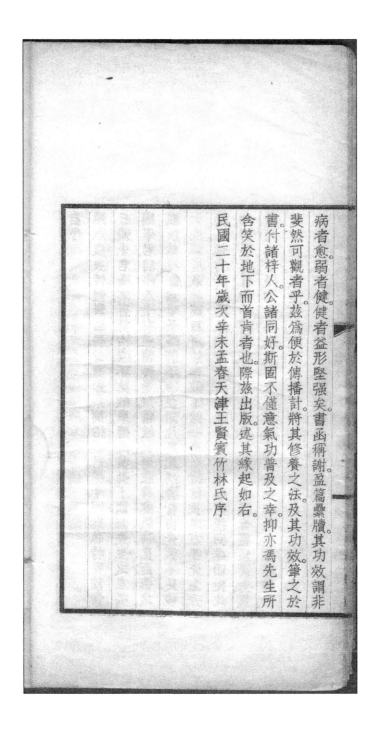

王竹林七十六小像

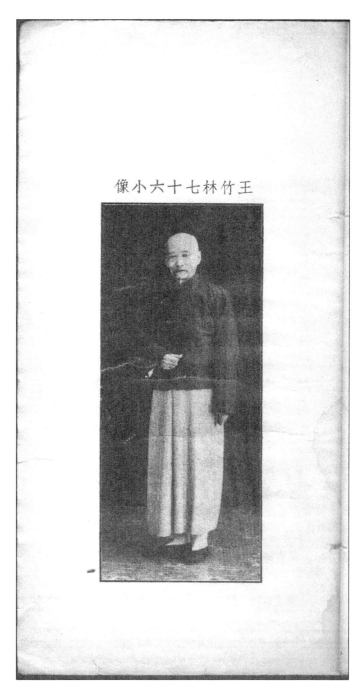

The author, Wang Zhu-lin

正面姿勢

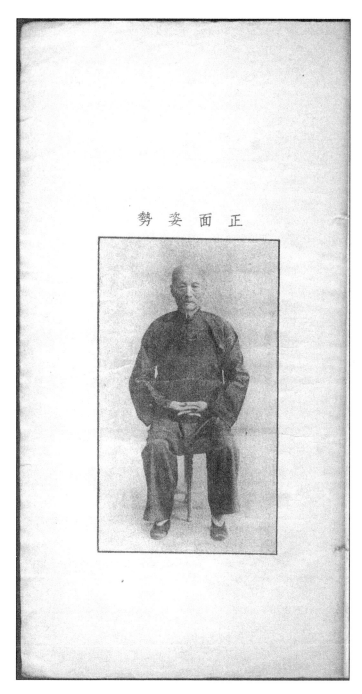

Wang Zhu-lin demonstrates the posture of tranquil sitting

側面姿勢

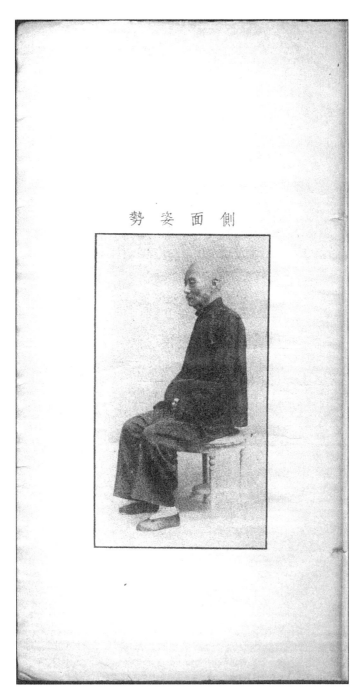

Wang Zhu-lin demonstrates the posture of tranquil sitting

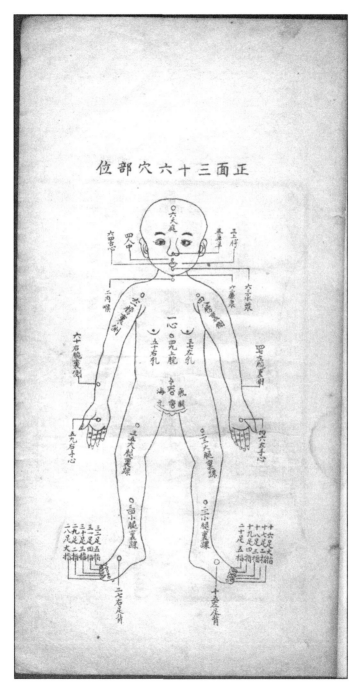

The locations of the 64 acupoints of the Intention and Qi Exercise

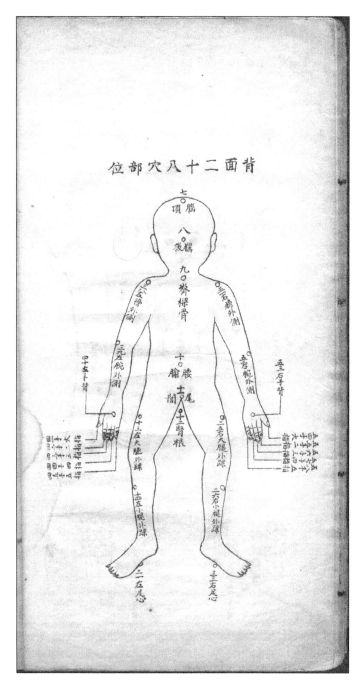

The locations of the 64 acupoints of the Intention and Qi Exercise

CHAPTER 1

The Beginnings of Health Cultivation

In general, when the men and the women, the old and the young are suffering with disease, [it is mainly because] unnoticed and lurking among the channels, and all through the 64 acupoints, [there is a large build-up of] qi depression and blood stasis which has accumulated over a long period of time.

When the disease arrives, if it is not serious, it can be treated with the [correct] diagnosis and treatment, but if it is severe no medicine or healing stone can reach it. If wishing to treat [the disease] with the Tao of the Heavenly Orbit, and moving the qi and blood through practicing Yi Qi Gong (Intention and Qi exercise), then every day, sincerely and meticulously, you should dedicate some time for training. Or you can strictly practice once, in the early morning, when the channels and collaterals of the whole body are dredged and feel comfortable. Within 100 days you can obtain an effect. When he was young, Yue Wu-mu (i.e. General Yue Fei) of the Song Dynasty was studying at the Da Fo Temple in Tangyin. [At the time] his body was weak and had many diseases. Therefore the Abbot Ci Hui, who was a Zen Master, bestowed to him this art. [After meticulous practice] his body was strengthened and all the diseases disappeared. Later he allowed this art to be handed down to others. If practiced sincerely for all of one's life, you can regulate the qi and nourish the blood, and [then] all disease will be cured and disappear. With personal efforts one can attain long life.

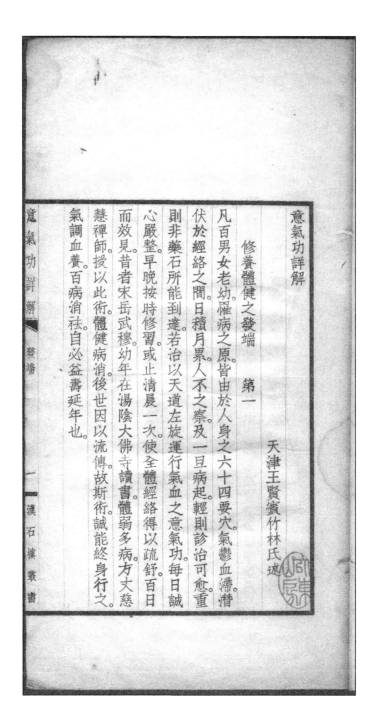

意氣功詳解

修養體健之發端　第一

天津王賢賓竹林氏述

凡百男女老幼罹病之原皆由於人身之六十四要穴氣鬱血滯潛
伏於經絡之間日積月累人不之察及一旦病起輕則診治可愈重
則非藥石所能到達若治以天道左旋運行氣血之意氣功每日誠
心嚴整早晚按時修習或止清晨一次使全體經絡得以疏舒百日
而效見昔者宋岳武穆幼年在湯陰大佛寺讀書體弱多病方丈慧
慧禪師授以此術體健病消後世因以流傳故斯術誠能終身行之
氣調血養百病消袪自必益壽延年也

意氣功詳解　發端
一
漢石樓叢書

CHAPTER 2

The Course of Training the Yi Qi Gong Exercise

Every morning, before washing, rinse your mouth with slightly salted water to remove the turbid qi of the mouth [and then start the exercise].

Sit on a short chair. You don't have to be restrained [by any complicated principles], but just assume a natural posture. The upper body, thighs and lower legs must be on a straight line.[1] The toes are bending slightly towards the inside. The eyes are closed to congeal the spirit. The hands are crossed over the Qi Hai (CV-6) point (Sea of Qi). Close the mouth and breathe in and out three times through your nose. Close the eyes, [and the head should be] facing straight. The tip of the tongue is slightly touching the palate.

Concentrate in order to congeal the spirit. Try to keep down any random thoughts. Out of the emptiness imagine the qi of the whole body gathering together just above the heart, and binding [it] into becoming a ball. Concentrate on this ball.

1. The starting point is the heart.

2. Ascend up to the throat.

3. Travel to the palate.

---

1 As a rule of thumb, when you sit the feet should be shoulder-width apart, and the shoulders, knees and feet should be on a straight line.

練習意氣之課程　第二

練習者應每日晨起暫不梳洗先以淡鹽湯漱口除去口中濁氣然後端坐矮椅不必矜持作態應取自然姿勢上身及大腿小腿三部皆宜平直兩足指部稍向內閉目凝神兩手交叉以抵氣海合口以鼻呼吸各三次開目平視舌尖微抵上膛。

壹志凝神力抑雜念憑空設一意想要使我週身之氣團聚心上結成一球復想此球。

一　由心起點

二　上行至咽喉

三　行至上膛、

4. Then move to the Ren Zhong (GV-26) point (human center).

5. Travel up to the Bi Zhun (GV-25) point (tip of the nose).

6. Then move [the ball] to the center of the forehead.

7. And travel to the top of the head.

8. Change the direction towards the back of the head.

9. And slowly move downwards to the spine.

10. And travel to the Yao Shu (GV-2) point (Lumbar Shu).

11. Then move [the ball] down to the coccyx.

12. And travel forwards to the kidney root (GV-1).

13. And then turn towards the lateral side of the left thigh (lit. towards the external malleolus).

14. And downwards to the lateral side of the left crus (lit. towards the external malleolus).

四　行至人中

五　行至鼻準

六　行至天庭

七　行至腦頂

八　轉行至腦後

九　徐徐下行至脊樑骨

十　行至腰腧

十一　下行至尾閭

十二　前行至腎根

十三　左行至左大腿外踝

十四　下行至左小腿外踝

15. Traveling to the dorsum of the left foot.

16. And continue down to the big toe of the left foot.

17. Then to the second toe.

18. And the third toe.

19. And the fourth toe.

20. And the fifth toe.

21. Then moving towards the Zu Xin point (Sole Heart).

22. Ascend through the medial side of the left crus (lit. starting from the internal malleolus).

23. Continue [upwards] across the medial side of the left thigh (lit. from the internal malleolus).

24. And ascend to the Guan Yuan point (CV-4).

25. Then to the right side, across the lateral side of the right thigh (lit. towards the external malleolus).

十五　行至左足背
十六　行至左足大指
十七　行至左足二指
十八　行至左足三指
十九　行至左足四指
二十　行至左足五指
二一　折至左足心
二二　上行至左小腿裏踝
二三　上行至左大腿裏踝
二四　上行至關元
二五　右行至右大腿外踝

175

26. And downwards to the lateral side of the right crus (lit. towards the external malleolus).

27. And continue to the dorsum of the right foot.

28. Move [the ball] to the big toe of the right foot.

29. And then to the second toe.

30. And the third toe.

31. And the fourth toe.

32. And the fifth toe.

33. And roll over to the Zu Xin [Yong Quan] point (KI-1) (Sole Heart).

34. Ascend up across the medial side of the right crus (lit. starting from the internal malleolus).

35. And across the medial side of the right thigh (lit. from the internal malleolus).

36. And ascend to the Qi Hai point (CV-6).

二六　下行至右小腿外踝

二七　行至右足背

二八　行至右足大指

二九　行至右足二指

三十　行至右足三指

三一　行至右足四指

三二　行至右足五指

三三　折至右足心

三四　上行至右小腿裏踝

三五　行至右大腿裏踝

三六　上行至氣海

177

37. Then [upwards] to the left breast.

38. Move across the outer side of the left shoulder.

39. And downwards towards the lateral side of the left wrist.

40. And traveling across the back of the left hand.

41. And then to the thumb of the left hand.

42. And then the pointing finger.

43. Then the middle finger.

44. Then the ring finger.

45. And the little finger.

46. And move to the center of the hand.

47. And up to the medial side of the left wrist.

三七　行至左乳

三八　左行至左肩膀外側

三九　下行至左手腕外側

四十　行至左手背

四一　行至左手大指

四二　行至左手二指

四三　行至左手三指

四四　行至左手四指

四五　行至左手五指

四六　行至左手心

四七　上行至左手腕裏側

48. And continue to the medial side of the left shoulder.

49. And travel to the middle of the stomach duct.

50. Move to the right breast.

51. And then to the lateral side of the right shoulder.

52. Travel to the outer side of the right wrist.

53. And move to the back of the right hand.

54. And then the right thumb.

55. The right pointing finger.

56. The middle finger.

57. The ring finger.

58. And the little finger.

四八　行至左肩膊裏側

四九　行至脘中

五十　行至右乳

五一　右行至右肩膊外側

五二　行至右手腕外側

五三　行至右手背

五四　行至右手大指

五五　行至右手二指

五六　行至右手三指

五七　行至右手四指

五八　行至右手五指

59. Move to the center of the hand.

60. And upwards to the medial side of the right hand.

61. And to the inner side of the right shoulder.

62. And then the Lian Quan (CV-23) Ridge Spring point.

63. Continue to the Cheng Jiang (CV-24) Sauce Receptacle point.

64. Then the center of the tongue and return to the heart.

At that point, the mouth will be full of liquids. Do not swallow yet. With the tongue flat, tap your teeth 36 times. After the liquids have already become frothy from the tapping, swallow them down in one gulp. Again close your mouth and breathe in and out three times through the nose. Slowly stand up with your hands dropping softly by the side. Gently move seven steps forwards. Go back and forth for seven steps for seven times. The exercise standard is that it should be completed in about ten minutes.

The act of binding the qi into a ball and moving it around entirely by the power of the Yi (intention) belongs to the Taoist methodology of training the qi to become elixir.

五九　行至右手心

六十　上行至右手腕裏側

六一　行至右肩膀裏側

六二　行至廉泉

六三　行至承漿

六四　行至舌心順行回至心部

此時口中津液已滿切勿咽下將舌放平叩齒三十六響津液因叩成沫一氣咽下再合口以鼻呼吸各三次稍定起立雙手下垂向前徐行七步爲一次。往來七次。功畢約以十分鐘爲標準。

夫所謂聚氣結球行至某處者全屬以意設想此即修道家煉氣成丹之要法也。

183

CHAPTER 3

Preventing and Eliminating Diseases

In the past, the daily Taoist health cultivation was mainly entrusted [to others while] written in an elusive way. Nobody could study or research it, or explain how the creator came to develop [these exercises], but merely [learnt about] how these exercises were transmitted [from teacher to disciple]. [One was supposed to] set up the altar, give and receive, respectfully undergo the ceremonial washing and [then] be included among the disciples, [often] even having to swear an oath to preserve the secrets. Because [of so much etiquette] and so many rules to consider, there was hesitation to reveal anything.

Only the Yi Qi Gong exercise, which is fully explained here, is presented without any secrecy, alongside its entire imagery and visualizations, and with its spirit being completely based on mental activities.

[Imagine] as if there is a line of spirit qi, starting from the heart and moving along with [the power of] thought, passing through 64 areas. These are the most important acupoints of the entire body [and the imbalance of] each of which is related with the development of a specific disease. If one practices on a daily basis, the psychological effects of the spirit will penetrate and infuse all the various points, the qi and blood will flow smoothly, and all disease will be eliminated through prevention of its development. Here is therefore provided a list of all the acupoints where the qi should circulate by the power of Yi (intention), and the relationship [of these points] with disease, one by one as follows:

意氣功詳解

預消疾病之功效　第三

在昔修道養生大抵托言神秘莫可究詰不曰某祖所創卽曰某師
所傳設壇授受必先恭行洗禮列入弟子甚至宣誓謹守秘密而一
般懷疑之士不免爲之逡巡却顧也惟茲所載之意氣功悉去神秘
之說專示其實際所謂假設意想全屬心理作用精神所到彷彿有
一線精氣隨心之所思而運行其經過之六十四部又爲全身之要
穴皆關係各病所自發吾人若日日利用其心理作用精神貫注遍
及各穴氣血通暢疾病卽消於未發之先矣茲將意氣所運行各部
之穴及關係疾病分別縷述如左。

意氣功詳解　功效

一

漢石樓叢書

185

1. **Heart:** The heart is the ruler of the body, and the path to life and death. The heart engenders all kinds of desires. If the heart is quiet, all desires will also be quiet. Old friends often find it appropriate to do tranquil sitting meditation, and repeatedly adjust the heart and the breath-qi [with] the two eyes loose like curtains that mirror the inner reflection. [And] descending the heart fire down to the dan tian, making their spirit and qi mutually interlock. [Imbalance of the heart] relates to [the development of] hemiplegia, abstraction of the heart qi, mania, forgetfulness, cough and vomiting blood, sobbing and anguish, deficiency of heart qi in children, not talking for several years, and various other syndromes.

2. **Throat:** This is the larynx. [Its imbalance] relates to [the development of] throat impediment and dryness, painful and swollen throat, loss of voice, inability to swallow water, and similar syndromes.

3. **Palate:** Inside the mouth, the center of the palate (Duan Jiao (GV-28) Extremity Intersection Point). [It can treat] pitting sores on the nose, red face and heart vexation, dry teeth with swollen and painful [gums], cold and summer heat scourge epidemic, and other syndromes.

一　心

心乃一身主宰生死路頭心生則種種欲生心靜則種種欲
靜故人常宜靜坐燕居調心息氣兩目垂簾返光內照心
火於丹田使神氣相抱也關係半身不遂心氣恍惚狂走健
忘欬吐血語泣悲小兒心氣不足數歲不語等症。

二　咽喉

內喉卽喉嚨關係喉凍乾燥咽喉腫痛喉喘不能言水粒不
下等症。

三　上腭

口中上腭中間爲（齗交穴）關係鼻中蝕瘡面赤心煩牙
疳腫痛寒暑瘟疫等症。

4. **Ren Zhong (GV-26), human center:** Alternatively known as the Shui Gou (water through) point. [It can treat] dispersion thirst (wasting and thirsting), excessive drinking of water, generalized puffy swelling, withdrawal and epilepsy, abnormal laughing and weeping, and other syndromes.

5. **Bi Zhun (GV-25), tip of the nose:** The ending of the nose pillar is alternatively called the Su Liao (white bone hole) point. This is the point of both exit and entry of the nasal passage. [It can treat] excessive nasal mucus, eruption of sores, nosebleed, and various other syndromes.

6. **Tian Ting, center of the forehead:** Half-way between the hairline and the nose, this is also called the Shen Ting (GV-24) Spirit Court point. [It can treat] mania and withdrawal, looking at but not recognizing people, dizzy vision due to head wind, clear nasal mucus, fright palpitations, and other syndromes.

7. **Top of the head:** This is also called the Bai Hui (GV-20) Hundred Convergences point. [It can treat] loss of voice after stroke, abstraction of the heart spirit, insanity and withdrawal, uncontrollably speaking anything that comes into the mind, headache and dizzy vision, and other syndromes.

四　人中

人中爲（水溝穴）。關係消渴飲水無度。水氣遍身浮腫癲
癇哭笑無常等症。

五　鼻準

鼻柱上端爲（素髎穴）。與肺經相表裏關係鼻中多瘜生
瘡鼻衄等症。

六　天庭

鼻上髮際五分爲（神庭穴）。關係癲狂目上視不識人頭
風目眩鼻出清涕驚悸等症。

七　腦頂

頂中爲（百會穴）。關係中風口禁心神恍惚風癇言語不

8. **Back of the head:** The back of the head is located one inch from the hairline, that is, the Feng Fu (GV-16) Wind House point. [Its imbalance] is related to [the development of] wind stroke, general heaviness and the neck not being able to turn, throat pain due to cold injury, and other syndromes.

9. **Spine:** This is the first disc of the spine Da Zhui (GV-14) Great Hammer point. [It can treat] distension of the lung, chest and rib-side fullness, abnormal rising of qi with vomiting, five kinds of strain[1] and seven injuries,[2] chest bind, and other syndromes.

10. **Yao Shu:** The Yao Shu (GV-2) point [is] the depression under the 21st vertebra. [It can treat] lumbar and hip pain, inability to bend forwards and backwards, menstrual irregularity in women, and other syndromes.

11. **Coccyx:** The bone at the end of the sacral spine is the Chang Qiang (GV-1) Long Strong point. [It can treat] intestinal wind, hemorrhoids and fistula, lumbar spine pain, constipation and urinary difficulty, heavy-headedness and thorough-flux diarrhea, and other syndromes.

---

1   Looking, lying, sitting, standing or walking for a very long time.

2   Injury due to food, anxiety, drink, sexual intemperance, hunger, taxation and channel network and construction defense damage.

擇頭痛目眩等症。

八　腦後

腦後髮際一寸爲（風府穴）關係中風身重項不得轉咽

喉疼痛傷寒等症。

九　脊櫟骨

脊骨第一節爲（大椎穴）以下關係肺脹脇滿嘔吐上氣。

五癆七傷結胸等症。

十　腰腧

左右腰間爲（腰腧穴）二十一椎下宛宛中關係腰胯疼

痛不得俯仰婦人月經不調等症。

十一　尾閭

12. **Kidney root:** [Located] in the middle between the two lower Yin orifices [is] the Hui Yin (CV-1) Meeting of Yin point. [It can treat] itching inside the anal canal with chronic hemorrhoids, headache due to Yin pattern, irregular menstruation in women, and other syndromes.

13. **Lateral side of left thigh:** 6 cun above the knee is the Fu Tu (ST-32) Crouching Rabbit point. [It can treat] wind, consumption (tuberculosis), impediment and counterflow, hand and foot contracture, cold and numbness in the knees, inner thigh sinew and collaterals' inability to bend and stretch, and other syndromes.

14. **Lateral side of the left crus:** 3 cun below the knee is the Zu San Li (ST-36) Leg-Three-Li point. [It can treat] deficiency cold of the stomach, counterflow of qi in the abdomen, thunderous rumbling in the intestines, knee and shin soreness and ache, and other syndromes.

脊骶骨端為（長强穴。）關係腸風痔瘻腰脊疼痛。大小便秘。頭重洞泄等症。

十二　腎根

囊底兩陰之間為（會陰穴。）關係穀道搔癢久痔相通。陰症頭痛及女子月經失時等症。

十三　左大腿外踝

膝上六寸為（伏兔穴。）關係風勞痺逆手足攣縮膝寒不仁。股內筋絡不屈伸等症。

十四　左小腿外踝

膝下三寸為（三里穴。）關係胃中虛寒。腹有逆氣腸如雷鳴。膝脛痠痛等症。

15. **Dorsum of the left foot:** 5 cun above the tarsus is the Chong Yang (ST-42) Surging Yang point. [It can treat] swelling and pain of the tarsus, distension and hardness of the abdomen, no pleasure in eating and drinking, climbing to high places and singing, casting off one's clothes and running around, and other syndromes.

16. **Big toe of the left foot:** This is the Da Dun (LV-1) Large Pile point. [It can treat] the five stranguries,[3] mounting qi, smaller abdomen (xiao fu) pain, somnolence, as well as all [patterns] related to Yin [pathology], and other syndromes.

17. **Second toe of the left foot:** Two points [are located here], the Li Dui (ST-45) Severe Mouth point and the Nei Ting (ST-44) Inner Court point. [They can treat] lockjaw, edema, cold malaria and wishing to lie down, reverse flow of the limbs, abdominal distension and fullness, and other syndromes.

18. **Third toe of the left foot:** This does not pertain to a principal acupuncture point and there isn't a [main] channel or collateral going through. However, in Yi Qi Gong [the qi] needs to circulate through that area too.

---

3   Stone, qi, unctuous, taxation and blood strangury.

足跗上五寸爲（衝陽穴）關係足跗腫痛肚腹堅大不嗜飲食登高而歌棄衣而走等症。

十六　左足大指

足大指端爲（大敦穴）關係五淋疝氣小腹疼痛喜寐以及陰中一切等症。

十七　左足二指

指端爲（厲兌內庭二穴）關係口禁水腫寒瘧好臥四肢厥逆肚腹脹滿等症。

十八　左足三指

此指無穴故不通經絡以意行氣時亦要行到。

19. **Fourth toe of the left foot:** This is the Qiao Yin[4] (GB-44) Orifice Yin point. [It can treat] rib-side pain, cough and counterflow, vexing heat in the hands and feet, stiff tongue and dry mouth, carbuncle and abscess, headache, and other syndromes.

20. **Fifth toe of the left foot:** This includes two points, the Zhi Yin (BL-67) Reaching Yin point and the Tong Gu (BL-66) Valley Passage point. [They can treat] eye screen and nasal congestion, cramps in cold malaria, dizzy vision and susceptibility to fright, cold injury with lack of sweat, and other syndromes.

21. **Left Zu Xin (Sole Heart) point:** The Sole Heart is the Yong Quan (KI-1) Gushing Spring point. [It can treat] left and right leg pain, irascibility and fearfulness, swollen throat and dry tongue, qi ascent heart vexation, all kinds of heat disease, and other syndromes.

22. **Medial side of the left crus:** 3 cun above the medial malleolus is the San Yin Jiao (SP-6) Three Yin Intersection point. [It can treat] weakness and deficiency of the spleen and stomach, distension and fullness in the heart and abdomen, kidney, liver and spleen channel disharmonies, and other syndromes.

---

4   The original text says Qiao Yang.

十九　左足四指

指端爲（竅陰穴）關係脇痛欬逆手足煩熱舌强口乾癰
疽頭痛等症。

二十　左足五指

指端爲（至陰通谷二穴）關係目翳鼻塞轉筋寒瘧目眩
善驚傷寒無汗等症。

二一　左足心

足心爲（湧泉穴）關係左右腿痛善恐惕惕咽腫舌乾上
氣心煩一切熱疾等症。

二二　左小腿裏踝

內踝上三寸爲（三陰交穴）關係脾胃虛弱心腹脹滿腎

197

23. **Medial side of the left thigh:** Medial to groin and on the fish belly [border] there is the Ji Men (SP-11) Winnower Gate point. [It can treat] qi counterflow, abdominal distension, urinary stoppage, and other syndromes.

24. **Guan Yuan point (CV-4):** 3 cun below the umbilicus is the Guan Yuan (CV-4) Pass Head point. [It can treat] gripping pain below the umbilicus, seminal emission with white turbidity, five stranguries, running piglet, accumulated cold deficiency fatigue, and other syndromes.

25. **Lateral side of the right thigh:** 6 cun above the knee is the Fu Tu (ST-32) Crouching Rabbit point. [It can treat] wind taxation, impediment and counterflow, hand and foot contracture, cold and numbness in the knees, inner thigh sinew and collaterals' inability to bend and stretch, and other syndromes.

26. **Lateral side of the right crus:** 3 cun below the knee is the Zu San Li (ST-36) Leg-Three-Li point. [It can treat] deficiency cold of the stomach, counterflow of qi in the abdomen, thunderous rumbling in the intestines, knee and shin soreness and ache, and other syndromes.

肝脾三經發現等症。

二三　左大腿裏踝

陰股內魚腹上越筋間為（箕門穴）關係氣逆腹脹。小便不通等症。

二四　關元

臍下三寸為（關元穴）關係臍下絞痛遺精白濁五淋黃豚積冷虛乏等症。

二五　右大腿外踝

膝上六寸為（伏兔穴）關係風勞痹逆手足攣縮膝寒不仁股內筋絡不能屈伸等症。

二六　右小腿外踝

27. **Dorsum of the right foot:** 5 cun above the tarsus is the Chong Yang (ST-42) Surging Yang point. [It can treat] swelling and pain of the tarsus, distension and hardness of the abdomen, no pleasure in eating and drinking, climbing to high places and singing, casting off one's clothes and running around, and other syndromes.

28. **Big toe of the right foot:** This is the Da Dun (LV-1) Large Pile point. [It can treat the development of] the five stranguries, mounting qi, smaller abdomen (xiao fu) pain, somnolence, as well as all [patterns] related to Yin [pathology], and other syndromes.

29. **Second toe of the right foot:** This includes two points, the Li Dui (ST-45) Severe Mouth point and the Nei Ting (ST-44) Inner Court point. [They can treat] lockjaw, edema, cold malaria and wishing to lie down, reverse flow of the limbs, abdominal distension and fullness, and other syndromes.

膝下三寸爲（三里穴）關係胃中虛寒腹有逆氣腸如雷
鳴膝脛痠痛等症。

二七　右足背

足跗上五寸爲（衝陽穴）關係足跗腫痛肚腹堅大不嗜
飲食登高而歌棄衣而走等症。

二八　右足大指

足大指端爲（大敦穴）關係五淋疝氣小腹疼痛喜寐以
及陰中一切等症。

二九　右足二指

指端爲（厲兌內庭二穴）關係口禁水腫寒瘧好臥四肢
厥逆肚腹脹滿等症。

201

30. **Third toe of the right foot:** This does not pertain to a [principal] acupuncture point and there isn't a [main] channel or collateral going through. However, in Yi Qi Gong [the qi] needs to circulate through that area too.

31. **Fourth toe of the right foot:** This is the Qiao Yin[5] GB-44 Orifice Yin point. [It can treat] rib-side pain, cough and counterflow, vexing heat in the hands and feet, stiff tongue and dry mouth, carbuncle and abscess, headache, and other syndromes.

32. **Fifth toe of the right foot:** This includes two points, the Zhi Yin (BL-67) Reaching Yin point and the Tong Gu (BL-66) Valley Passage point. [They can treat] eye screen and nasal congestion, cramps in cold malaria, dizzy vision and susceptibility to fright, cold injury with lack of sweat, and other syndromes.

33. **Right Zu Xin (Sole Heart) point:** The Sole Heart is the Yong Quan (KI-1) Gushing Spring point. [It can treat] left and right leg pain, irascibility and fearfulness, swollen throat and dry tongue, qi ascent heart vexation, all kinds of heat disease, and other syndromes.

---

5   The original text says Qiao Yang.

三十　右足三指

此指無穴。故不通經絡。以意行氣時亦要行到。

二九　右足四指

指端為（竅陰穴）。關係脇痛欬逆手足煩熱舌強口乾癧疽頭痛等症。

二八　右足五指

指端為（至陰通谷二穴）。關係目翳鼻塞轉筋寒瘧目眩善驚傷寒無汗等症。

二七　右足心

足心為（湧泉穴）。關係左右腿痛善恐惕惕咽腫舌乾上氣心煩一切熱疾等症。

203

34. **Medial side of the right calf:** 3 cun above the medial malleolus is the San Yin Jiao (SP-6) Three Yin Intersection point. [It can treat] weakness and deficiency of the spleen and stomach, distension and fullness in the heart and abdomen, kidney, liver and spleen channel disharmonies, and other syndromes.

35. **Medial side of the right thigh:** Medial to groin and on the fish belly [border] there is the Ji Men (SP-11) Winnower Gate point. [It can treat] qi counterflow, abdominal distension, urinary stoppage, and other syndromes.

36. **Qi Hai:** 1.5 cun below the umbilicus is the Qi Hai (CV-6) Sea of Qi point. It is the sea of qi generation in men, and the temple of childbearing in women. [It can treat] qi exhaustion and panting, and other syndromes.

37. **Center of the left breast:** The center of the breast is the Ru Zhong (ST-17) Breast Center point. [It can treat] nodes in the breast, breast paralysis (related to milk production), and breast furuncle. In women, [also] phlegm stagnation in the diaphragm, breast milk stoppage, and other syndromes.

三四　右小腿裏踝

內踝上三寸爲（三陰交穴）。關係脾胃虛弱心腹脹滿腎
肝脾三經發現等症。

三五　右大腿裏踝

陰股內魚腹上越筋間爲（箕門穴）。關係氣逆腹痛小便
不通等症。

三六　氣海

臍下一寸五分爲（氣海穴）。男子生氣之海。婦人生育之
關關係氣憊氣喘等症。

三七　左乳中

當乳正中爲（乳中穴）。關係乳中結核乳癰乳癧以及婦

205

38. **Outer side of the left shoulder:** At the end of the shoulder, in the middle of the two bones, is the Jian Yu (LI-15) Shoulder Bone point. [It can treat] sinew and bone weakness, shoulder and arm pain, wind heat dormant papules, color dry and withered, and other syndromes.

39. **Lateral side of the left wrist:** Below the curve of the radius and at the transverse crease of the elbow is located the Qu Chi (LI-11) Pool at the Bend point. [It can treat] redness and swelling of the arm, evil qi cold injury, flaky skin and itching, absence of menses, and other syndromes.

40. **Back of the left hand:** At the center of the back of the four metacarpal bones is the Zhong Zhu (TB-3) Central Islet point. [It can treat] heat syndromes, headaches, dizzy vision, tinnitus, elbow, arm, hand and finger pain, and other syndromes.

41. **Left thumb:** At the end of the left thumb is located the Shao Shang (LU-11) Lesser Shang point. [It can treat] mouth swelling, throat obstruction, sweating and feeling cold, cough and counterflow, phlegm malaria, [alternating] cold and heat, chattering of jaws, blockage of the throat, inability to swallow water and grains, and other syndromes.

人膈有滯痰乳汁不通等症。

三八　左膊外側

肩端上兩骨間爲（肩髃穴）關係筋骨無力肩臂疼痛風熱癧疹顏色枯焦等症。

三九　左腕外側

肘下輔骨曲肘橫紋頭爲（曲池穴）關係手臂紅腫邪氣傷寒皮脫作癢婦人月經不通等症。

四十　左手背

四指本節後陷中爲（中渚穴）關係熱症頭痛目眩耳聾。

四一　左手大指

肘臂手指疼痛等症。

42. **Left pointing finger:** In the medial side of the end of the [pointing] finger is the Shang Yang (LI-1) point. [It can treat] qi fullness in the chest, cough, swelling of the limbs, dry mouth, tinnitus, toothache, aversion to cold, and other syndromes.

43. **Left middle finger:** In the tip of the finger is the Zhong Chong (PC-9) Central Hub point. [It can treat] heat disease, vexation and oppression, absence of sweat, body heat like fire (fever), heart pain, vexation and fullness, stiff tongue, and other syndromes.

44. **Left ring finger:** At the tip is the Guang Chong (TB-1) Passage Hub point. [It can treat] throat blockage, curling of the tongue, headache, cholera, qi counterflow in the chest, pain and inability to lift the upper arm and elbow, and other syndromes.

手指端爲（少商穴）關係頷腫咽閉汗出而寒欬逆痰瘧。

寒熱鼓頷咽中閉塞水粒不下等症。

四二　左手二指

指端內側爲（商陽穴）關係胸中氣滿欬嗽肢腫口乾耳聾齒痛惡寒等症。

四三　左手三指

指端爲（中衝穴）關係熱病煩悶汗不得出身熱如火心痛煩滿舌强等症。

四四　左手四指

指端爲（關衝穴）關係咽閉舌捲頭痛霍亂胸中氣逆臂肘痛不可舉等症。

45. **Left little finger:** At the tip of the finger is the Shao Ze (SI-1) Lesser Marsh point. [It can treat] various types of malarial [alternating] heat and cold, heart vexation, dry mouth, cough, absence of sweat, nebulous eye screen relapse in the pupil of the eye, and other syndromes.

46. **Left hand center:** In the center of the palm is located the Lao Gong (PC-8) Palace of Toil point. [It can treat] wind stroke, irascibility, blood in the stool and urine, fishy smelling mouth, chest distension and rib-side fullness, inability to swallow food and drink, and other syndromes.

47. **Medial side of the left wrist:** 1.5 cun superior to the left wrist at the depression right under the index finger when [the thumbs and index fingers of] both hands are crossed is the location of the Lie Que (LU-7) Broken Sequence point. [It can treat] paralysis and swelling of the four extremities, bloody urine, seminal emission, and other syndromes.

48. **Medial side of the left shoulder:** Below the great bone is the Yun Men (LU-2) Cloud Gate point. [It can treat] chest and rib-side shortness of breath, incessant cough and counterflow, pain and inability to raise the forearm, binding and gathering of goiter, and other syndromes.

四五　左手五指

指端爲（少澤穴）關係諸瘧寒熱心煩口乾咳嗽無汗目生雲翳覆瞳子等症。

四六　左手心

掌中心爲（勞宮穴）關係中風善怒大小便血口中腥臭。

胸脹脇滿飲食不下等症。

四七　左腕裏側

腕側上一寸五分兩手交义食指盡處爲（列缺穴）關係

四肢癰腫弱血遺精等症。

四八　左膊裏側

巨骨下爲（雲門穴）關係胸脇氣短欬逆不息臂痛不舉。

211

49. **Upper stomach duct:** [Located here is the] Wei Wan (CV-12) Stomach Duct point, 5 cun superior to the umbilicus. [It can treat] non-transformation of food and drink, cholera vomiting and diarrhea, abdominal qi distension and fullness, heart agitation and fright palpitation, and other syndromes.

50. **Center of the right breast:** The center of the breast is the Ru Zhong (ST-17) Breast Center point. [It can treat] nodes in the breast, breast paralysis (related to milk production), and breast furuncle. In women, [also] phlegm stagnation in the diaphragm, breast milk stoppage, and other syndromes.

51. **Outer side of the right shoulder:** At the end of the shoulder, in the middle of the two bones, is the Jian Yu (LI-15) Shoulder Bone point. [It can treat] sinew and bone weakness, shoulder and arm pain, wind heat dormant papules, color dry and withered, and other syndromes.

52. **Lateral side of the right wrist:** Below the curve of the radius and at the transverse crease of the elbow is located the Qu Chi (LI-11) Pool at the Bend point. [It can treat] redness and swelling of the arm, evil qi cold injury, flaky skin and itching, absence of menses, and other syndromes.

癥氣結聚等症。

四九　上脘

一名（胃脘穴）臍上五寸關係水食不化霍亂吐瀉腹氣脹滿心忪驚悸等症。

五十　右乳中

當乳正中爲（乳中穴）關係乳中結核乳癰乳癖以及婦人膈有滯痰乳汁不通等症。

五一　右膀外側

肩端上兩骨間爲（肩髃穴）關係筋骨無力肩臂疼痛風熱癮疹顏色枯焦等症。

五二　右腕外側

213

53. **Back of the right hand:** At the center of the back of the four metacarpal bones is the Zhong Zhu (TB-3) Central Islet point. [It can treat] heat syndromes, headaches, dizzy vision, tinnitus, elbow, arm, hand and finger pain, and other syndromes.

54. **Right thumb:** At the end of the right thumb is located the Shao Shang (LU-11) Lesser Shang point. [It can treat] mouth swelling, throat obstruction, sweating and feeling cold, cough and counterflow, phlegm malaria, [alternating] cold and heat, chattering of jaws, blockage of the throat, inability to swallow water and grains, and other syndromes.

55. **Right pointing finger:** In the medial side of the end of the [pointing] finger is the Shang Yang (LI-1) point. [It can treat] qi fullness in the chest, cough, swelling of the limbs, dry mouth, tinnitus, toothache, aversion to cold, and other syndromes.

肘下輔骨曲肘横紋頭爲（曲池穴）。關係手臂紅腫邪氣
傷寒皮脱作癢婦人月經不通等症。

五三　右手背

四指本節後陷中爲（中渚穴）。關係熱症頭痛目眩耳聾。
肘臂手指疼痛等症。

五四　右手大指

手指端爲（少商穴）。關係頷腫咽閉汗出而寒欬
寒熱鼓頷咽中閉塞水粒不下等症。　逆痰瘧。

五五　右手二指

指端內側爲（商陽穴）。關係胸中氣滿咳嗽肢腫口乾耳
聾齒痛惡寒等症。

215

56. **Right middle finger:** In the tip of the finger is the Zhong Chong (PC-9) Central Hub point. [It can treat] heat disease, vexation and oppression, absence of sweat, body heat like fire (fever), heart pain, vexation and fullness, stiff tongue, and other syndromes.

57. **Right ring finger:** At the tip is the Guang Chong (TB-1) Passage Hub point. [It can treat] throat blockage, curling of the tongue, headache, cholera, qi counterflow in the chest, pain and inability to lift the upper arm and elbow, and other syndromes.

58. **Right little finger:** At the tip of the finger is the Shao Ze (SI-1) Lesser Marsh point. [It can treat] various types of malarial [alternating] heat and cold, heart vexation, dry mouth, cough, absence of sweat, nebulous eye screen relapse in the pupil of the eye, and other syndromes.

59. **Right hand center:** In the center of the palm is located the Lao Gong (PC-8) Palace of Toil point. [It can treat] wind stroke, irascibility, blood in the stool and urine, fishy smelling mouth, chest distension and rib-side fullness, inability to swallow food and drink, and other syndromes.

五六　右手二指

指端爲（中衝穴）。關係熱病煩悶汗不得出身熱如火心痛煩滿舌强等症。

五七　右手四指

指端爲（關衝穴）。關係喉閉舌捲頭痛霍亂胸中氣逆臂肘痛不可舉等症。

五八　右手五指

指端爲（少澤穴）。關係諸瘧寒熱心煩口乾咳嗽無汗目生雲翳覆瞳子等症。

五九　右手心

掌中心爲（勞宮穴）。關係中風善怒大小便血口中腥臭。

217

60. **Medial side of the right wrist:** 1.5 cun superior to the right wrist at the depression right under the index finger when [the thumbs and index fingers of] both hands are crossed is the location of the Lie Que (LU-7) Broken Sequence point. [It can treat] paralysis and swelling of the four extremities, bloody urine, seminal emission, and other syndromes.

61. **Medial side of the right shoulder:** Below the great bone is the Yun Men (LU-2) Cloud Gate point. [It can treat] chest and rib-side shortness of breath, incessant cough and counterflow, pain and inability to raise the forearm, binding and gathering of goiter, and other syndromes.

62. **Lian Quan:** Inferior to the nape, in the middle of the laryngeal prominence, is the Lian Quan (CV-23) Ridge Spring point, also known as She Ben (Tongue Root). [It can treat] cough, qi ascent, rapid panting, vomiting of froth, sudden retraction of the root of the tongue, and other syndromes.

63. **Cheng Jiang:** Inferior to the lip in the center of the mentolabial groove is the Cheng Jiang (CV-24) Sauce Receptacle point. [It can treat] hemilateral wind, teeth and mouth ulceration due to malnutrition, sudden loss of voice and speech, swelling of the face, Xiao Ke, and other syndromes.

胸脹脇滿飲食不下等症。

六十　右腕裏側

腕側上一寸五分兩手交叉食指盡處爲（列缺穴。）關係
四肢癰腫溺血遺精等症。

六一　右膀裏側

巨骨下爲（雲門穴）關係胸脇氣短欬逆不息臂痛不舉。

癭氣結聚等症。

六二　廉泉

項下結喉中間爲（廉泉穴）亦名舌本穴關係咳嗽上氣。

喘急嘔沫舌根縮急等症。

六三　承漿

64. **Center of the tongue:** At the center of the tongue is the Ju Quan (EX-HN-10) Gathering Spring point. [It can treat] tongue fur and tongue stiffness, sores inside the mouth, bone trough wind, double tongue swollen and distended, extreme heat and difficulty in speech, and other syndromes.

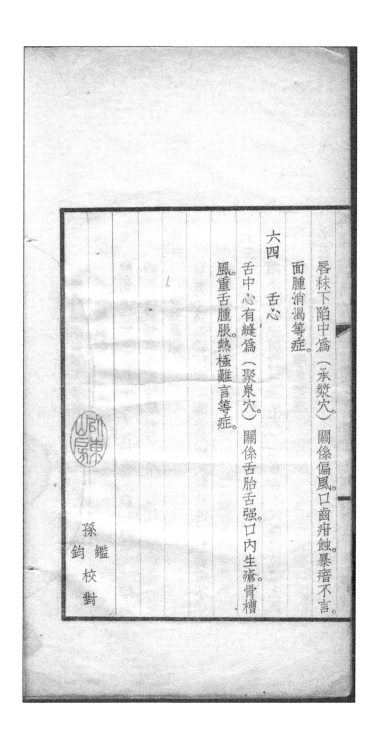

唇絍下陷中爲（承漿穴）關係偏風口齒舟蝕暴瘖不言。

面腫消渴等症。

六四　舌心

舌中心有縫爲（聚泉穴）關係舌胎舌強口內生瘡骨槽

風重舌腫脹熱極難言等症。

CHAPTER 4

"Intention and Qi Exercise" Instructions in Verse

I have practiced the "Intention and Qi Exercise" since I was a child, for more than 60 years and without any breaks. Over several decades I have instructed more than 1000 relatives and friends. The sick have been cured and the weak have become strong. The effects are so good that no words of praise are necessary. For promoting the method of cultivating this health exercise that can be used for preventing the development of disease, I have penned this book and made it public for all people. Recently many come to study, and during their daily practice they often forget the points or the course [of the movement]. [As a result] the students have expressed to me their difficulties in detail.

I feel ashamed for my blunt clumsiness. After practicing for many days, I am afraid that there were indeed some difficulties [in understanding] the first part of the book. This was unfortunate, and in view of this situation I examined the details and researched on how to supplement [this work]. I hope that all that engage in the study of this book will be successful. And hope that they can share its study and at the same time accomplish longevity. To answer their wish I here provide three poems that act as a shortcut [in the study of these materials]. The first is "The song for the movement of qi," the second is "The song for the six demands of the acupoints" and the third is "The song for the completion of the exercise."

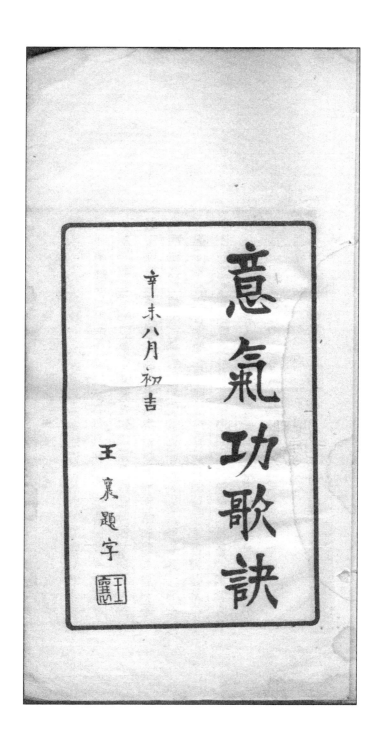

意氣功歌訣

辛未八月初吉

王襄題字

All who wish to recuperate their bodies first do not rush to practice. Devote your efforts to studying the *Detailed Exposition of the Intention and Qi Exercise*. Study repeatedly until you have memorized its contents. Then study the shortcut songs until you have mastered them. Do that before starting to practice. If you use the poems in your everyday study it will be easy to progress, being free from the anxiety of omitting parts of the exercise or fearing that it is difficult to practice. Then the progress from being a beginner to becoming a skilled practitioner will be smooth and unimpeded. Again examine all the details in the *Detailed Exposition*. The ball of qi that gathers together above the heart should enter the channels through the points and move with the power of the Yi (intention). Pay attention to the additional comments. Every day you should arrange a standard time of ten minutes for practicing.

意氣功歌訣

愚自幼修習意氣功迄今六十餘載。未嘗間斷。且此數十年中口授
戚友不下數十百人。病者愈健其功效。勿庸贅述愚爲提倡體
育計已將修養練習之法及預消疾病之功效筆之於書付諸梓人。
公諸同好。惟近日來學者甚夥。其中有每日練習時常將課程及各
穴部位忘記顛倒。而學者詳述困難自慚鈍拙以致練習數十日畏
難中輟爲可惜愚有鑑於此詳察情形研究補助方法希望所學
普及成就。並期轉相傳習同登壽域以償夙願茲特補註捷徑歌三
章。一運氣歌二六要穴歌三功畢歌凡有志修身者切勿急於練習
務將意氣功詳解之（自序）（發端）（課程）（功效）通篇
反覆細閱了然於胸中再將捷徑歌讀之純熟方可入手每日先按

意氣功詳解 補註 一二 漢石橫叢書

If [you are] determined, this practice can sincerely repair your body. If you keep practicing continuously for 100 days, you shall enter the realm of the Tao. For the scholars that look forwards to the results, the effect would be immediately evident. If one persistently pursues this for one's whole life, this exercise will help in eliminating disease and prolonging life. The information [offered here] is provided to scholars as a supplement to the previous materials.

Xin Wei year (1931), 7th lunar month, one
day after the Qi Qiao festival
Supplemented by Scholar Wang Zhu-lin
at the Han Shi Lou

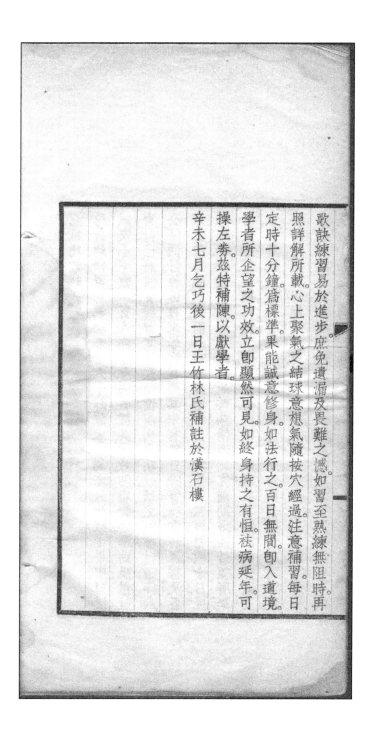

歌訣練習易於進步庶免遺漏及畏難之憾如習至熟練無阻時再
照詳解所載心上聚氣之結球意想氣隨按穴經過注意補習每日
定時十分鐘爲標準果能誠意修身如法行之百日無間即入道境。
學者所企望之功效立即顯然可見如終身持之有恆祛病延年可
操左券茲特補陳以獻學者。

辛未七月乞巧後一日王竹林氏補註於漢石樓

The song for the movement of qi

Sit naturally, the three divisions[1] balanced
The legs must bend[2] in the middle
Eyes closed, hands crossed
Crossed horizontal to the Qi Hai (CV-6) point (Sea of Qi)
Close the mouth and breathe in and out through the nose three times
Close the eyes, and the tip of the tongue softly touches the palate
Imagine that the qi from all over the body is gathering just above the
    heart
Binds into a ball and moves upwards

Each course, from sitting down, to imagining the qi, binding it into a ball and gathering above the heart, takes a total of 2 minutes.

The song for the six demands of the acupoints

From the heart ascend to the throat and circle to the root of the kidney
    (*The movement of qi, starting from the heart and arriving to the root
    of the kidney, should take 1 minute*)
From the kidney root move towards the left and loop back to the
    Guang Yuan point (*1 minute*)
From Guang Yuan move towards the right, then make a circle back to
    Qi Hai (*1 minute*)
From Qi Hai move towards the left breast and return to the stomach
    duct (*1 minute*)
From the stomach duct move towards the right breast and end up at
    the Lian Quan point (*1 minute*)
From Lian Quan return to the heart and the origin of the movement
    (*1 minute*)

Complete the above instructions after the ball binding above the heart. (*Move according to the six demands of the acupoints and return to the heart. This course should take 6 minutes.*)

---

1   Although here the three divisions should be understood as lower, middle and
     upper body, or lower leg, thigh and upper body (according to how one sits on a
     chair), it can also be further interpreted as the three internal and three external
     harmonies in balance.

2   Because obviously one is sitting on a chair.

運氣歌

端坐自然三部平　　須知兩足向中傾

閉目雙手交叉勢　　交叉微倚氣海橫

合口鼻孔三呼吸　　開目舌尖抵腭輕

週身氣想心頭集　　結合如球向上行

自端坐及各課程。至想氣結球。集於心頭。功用二分鐘。

六要穴歌

心起行喉轉腎根　　自心起運氣轉至腎根　　注意一分鐘

腎根向左繞關元　　由腎根繞氣繞至關元　　注意一分鐘

關元向右迴氣海　　由關元還氣迴至氣海　　注意一分鐘

氣海左乳脘中原　　由氣海運氣左至脘中　　注意一分鐘

The song for the completion of the exercise

Do not swallow the saliva that fills the mouth
With the tongue flat, tap the teeth beating the saliva
In one gulp swallow down to the dan tian
Breathe in and out three times through the nose
Stand up and both hands fall comfortably at the side
Go back and forth 7 steps for 7 times
In 100 days, if practiced without breaks, it will remove the disease
If you practice all of your life you can enjoy longevity

(*From the point where the saliva fills the mouth to walking 7 steps 7 times and the completion of the exercise, it takes 2 minutes*)

The three poems, as described above, detail the movement of the qi along the acupoints, until the completion of the exercise. You should practice every day. The whole procedure should take 10 minutes.

脘中右乳廉泉穴　由脘中運氣右至廉泉　注意一分鐘

廉泉回心返本源　由廉泉運氣回至心部　注意一分鐘

由心起之結球向上運行六要穴回至心。　功用六分鐘。

功畢歌

唾滿口中先勿咽　舌平叩齒攪成涎

一氣咽下丹田覺　三次呼吸鼻內含

雙足起立雙垂手　七步來回七次連

百日無間能除病　終身有恒享大年

由唾滿口中及各課程至七步七次功畢。　功用二分鐘。

以上由運氣行穴至功畢按三歌訣每日練習。　綜計十分鐘。

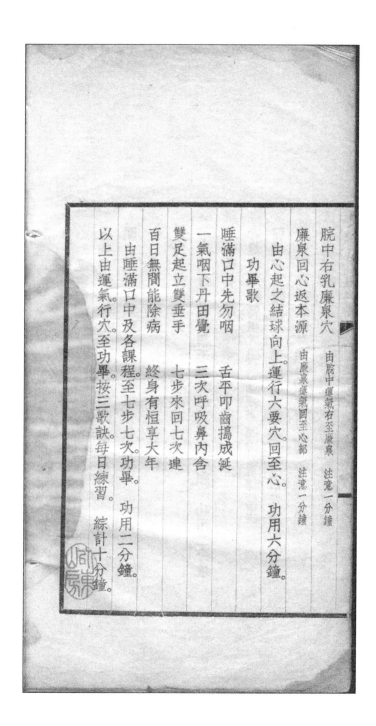

231

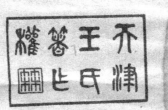

天津文嵐簃承印

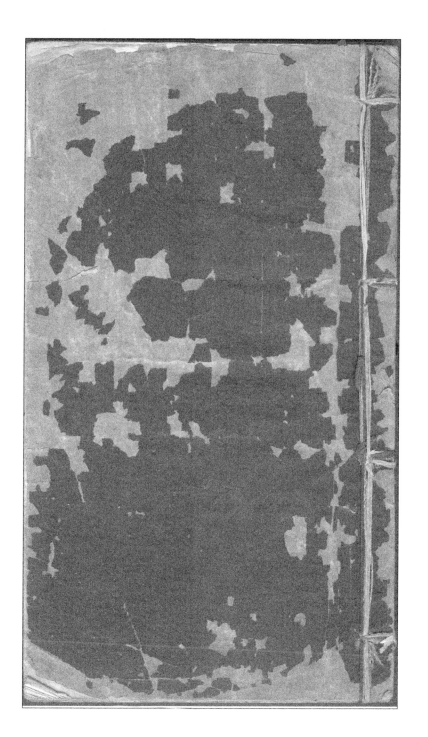

MASTER BU ENFU'S YI QUAN LINEAGE AND TRAINING METHODOLOGY

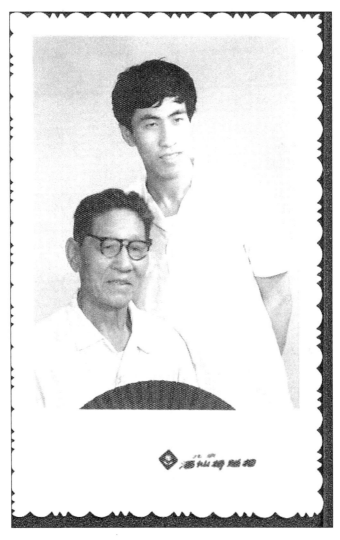

Master Bu Enfu with Cui Fushan

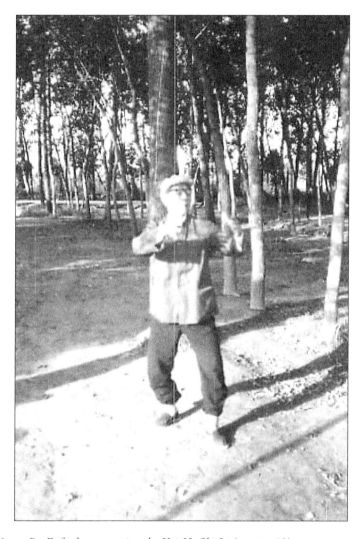

Master Bu Enfu demonstrating the Kai He Shi Li (exercise 12)

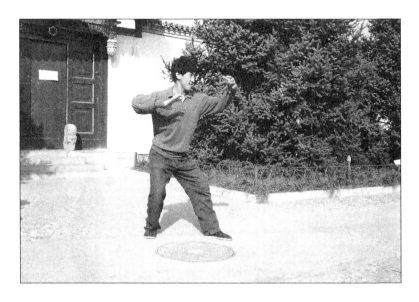

Master Cui Fushan demonstrating a variant of the Hun Yuan Zhuang (exercise 8, variant 2)

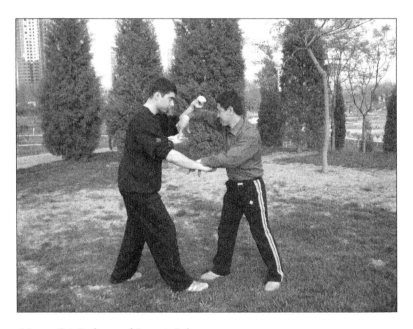

Master Cui Fushan and Ioannis Solos

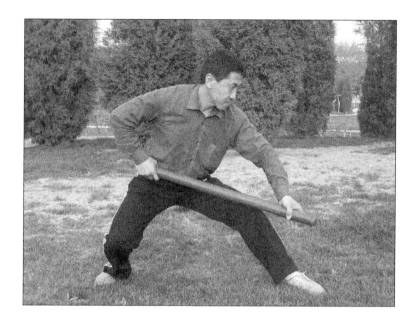

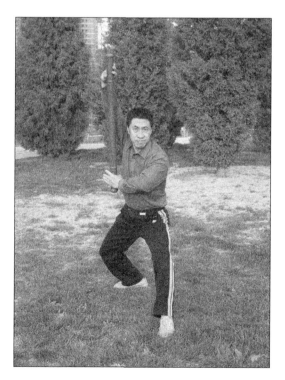

Master Cui Fushan demonstrating Yi Chuan Long Ruler exercises

THE COURSE OF THE QI IN THE INTENTION AND QI EXERCISE

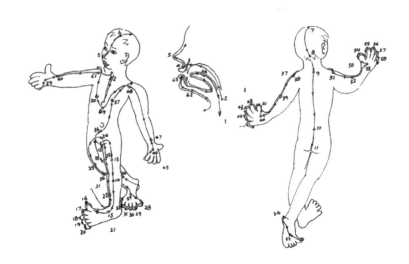

1.	Heart (no point)	12.	Hui Yin (CV-1)
2.	Throat (no point)	13.	Fu Tu (ST-32)
3.	Duan Jiao (GV-28)	14.	Zu San Li (ST-36)
4.	Ren Zhong (GV-26)	15.	Chong Yang (ST-42)
5.	Bi Zhun (GV-25)	16.	Da Dun (LV-1)
6.	Shen Ting (GV-24)	17.	Li Dui (ST-45) and Nei Ting (ST-44)
7.	Bai Hui (GV-20)		
8.	Feng Fu (GV-16)	18.	Middle toe (no point)
9.	Da Zhui (GV-14)	19.	Qiao Yin (GB-44)
10.	Yao Shu (GV 2)	20.	Zhi Yin (BL-67) and Tong Gu (BL-66)
11.	Chang Qiang (GV-1)		

21. Yong Quan (KI-1)
22. San Yin Jiao (SP-6)
23. Ji Men (SP-11)
24. Guan Yuan (CV-4)
25. Fu Tu (ST-32)
26. Zu San Li (ST-36)
27. Chong Yang (ST-42)
28. Da Dun (LV-1)
29. Li Dui (ST-45) and Nei Ting (ST-44)
30. Middle toe (no point)
31. Qiao Yin (GB-44)
32. Zhi Yin (BL-67) and Tong Gu (BL-66)
33. Yong Quan (KI-1)
34. San Yin Jiao (SP-6)
35. Ji Men (SP-11)
36. Qi Hai (CV-6)
37. Ru Zhong (ST-17)
38. Jian Yu (LI-15)
39. Qu Chi (LI-11)
40. Zhong Zhu (TB-3)
41. Shao Shang (LU-11)
42. Shang Yang (LI-1)
43. Zhong Chong (PC-9)
44. Guang Chong (TB-1)
45. Shao Ze (SI-1)
46. Lao Gong (PC-8)
47. Lie Que (LU-7)
48. Yun Men (LU-2)
49. Wei Wan (CV-12)
50. Ru Zhong (ST-17)
51. Jian Yu (LI-15)
52. Qu Chi (LI-11)
53. Zhong Zhu (TB-3)
54. Shao Shang (LU-11)
55. Shang Yang (LI-1)
56. Zhong Chong (PC-9)
57. Guang Chong (TB-1)
58. Shao Ze (SI-1)
59. Lao Gong (PC-8)
60. Lie Que (LU-7)
61. Yun Men (LU-2)
62. Lian Quan (CV-23)
63. Cheng Jiang (CV-24)
64. Ju Quan (EX-HN-10)

ABOUT THE AUTHOR

Ioannis Solos studied Traditional Chinese Medicine at Middlesex University and the Beijing University of Chinese Medicine. He enjoys researching, teaching, practicing and critically interpreting the ancient philosophy and culture of China, internal martial arts, health preservation practices, classic medical texts and lesser-known Chinese esoteric traditions. He is the author of *Gold Mirrors and Tongue Reflections*, also published by Singing Dragon.